Neurosurgery: Concerns and Issues

Neurosurgery: Concerns and Issues

Edited by **Arthur Colfer**

New Jersey

Published by Foster Academics,
61 Van Reypen Street,
Jersey City, NJ 07306, USA
www.fosteracademics.com

Neurosurgery: Concerns and Issues
Edited by Arthur Colfer

International Standard Book Number: 978-1-63242-287-3 (Hardback)

Printed in the United States of America.

Contents

Permissions

List of Contributors

Preface

Every book is a source of knowledge and this one is no exception. The idea that led to the conceptualization of this book was the fact that the world is advancing rapidly; which makes it crucial to document the progress in every field. I am aware that a lot of data is already available, yet, there is a lot more to learn. Hence, I accepted the responsibility of editing this book and contributing my knowledge to the community.

Neurosurgery is a field of medical study which is growing at a steady speed. Therefore, it is imperative for trainers, as well as neurosurgeons to keep themselves updated with new discoveries and developments occurring in this field. Functional neurosurgery, advanced techniques and hemostatic agents in neurosurgery are some of the topics discussed in the book. This book is an attempt to provide knowledge to all those who are interested in the field of neurosurgery.

While editing this book, I had multiple visions for it. Then I finally narrowed down to make every chapter a sole standing text explaining a particular topic, so that they can be used independently. However, the umbrella subject sinews them into a common theme. This makes the book a unique platform of knowledge.

I would like to give the major credit of this book to the experts from every corner of the world, who took the time to share their expertise with us. Also, I owe the completion of this book to the never-ending support of my family, who supported me throughout the project.

Editor

Section 1

Spinal Issues

Craniovertebral Junction Chordomas

Pratipal Kalsi and David Choi
National Hospital for Neurology & Neurosurgery, London
United Kingdom

1. Introduction

Chordomas are rare tumours that arise from remnants of the embryonic notochord. They can be located in all places where the notocord existed, such as the nasopharynx, clivus, sella turcica, foramen magnum, cervical spine and sacrococcygeal region. This chapter will focus on chordomas affecting the craniovertebral junction (CV). Chordomas are rare malignant tumours with an incidence of less than 1 per 100,000. The site of origin of skull base chordomas is usually the clivus and from here they can extend into the anterior fossa, middle fossa, the sellar and parasellar regions, and through the foramen magnum into the upper cervical spine. In the majority of cases the typical histological appearances and characteristic location of chordomas render the diagnosis straightforward. The symptoms and signs are highly variable and depend on the exact site of the lesion and the involvement of adjacent structures. These can range from cranial nerve palsies, motor and sensory deficits, to gait disturbance and balance problems. Radiological diagnosis of craniovertebral junction chordomas has improved with the advent of modern CT and MR imaging modalities and tumour location and extent of skull base involvement can be precisely defined. Surgery is the most effective form of treatment for patients with craniovertebral junction chordomas and radical resection augmented with adjuvant therapies such as proton beam therapy have been shown to prolong survival. Although chordomas are usually slow-growing tumours they are locally aggressive with a tendency to infiltrate adjacent tissues and organs. Local recurrence is common and often causes death. Metastasis is well documented but is uncommon. This chapter will aim to give an overview of the diagnosis and management of CV junction chordomas.

2. Epidemiology

Chordomas are rare tumours arising from persistent rests of notochordal remnants. They constitute 0.2% of all CNS tumours. Chordomas represent between 1% to 8% of primary malignant bone tumours and 20% of those arising from the spine. (Rosenberg AE, 2003) The age adjusted incidence for chordomas is 0.08 per 100 000.

There is a 2:1 male preponderance for all chordomas. However, CV junction chordomas have a more equal sex distribution. There is a strikingly low incidence in ethnic minorities and the incidence in African Americans is around quarter of that in white populations.

These tumours tend to occur across a wide age range and the peak incidence varies with anatomical location. Chordomas of the CV junction present more commonly during the fourth and fifth decades with the average age at diagnosis being 38 years. They generally present at a younger age than sacral and vertebral chordomas. In comparison, sacral chordomas tend to present at an older age, with the average age of presentation being 56 years.

Small series of childhood chordomas have been reported and these are usually found at the skull base. However, they account for less than 5% of all chordomas. Familial chordoma has been described but is extremely rare and several chromosomal loci have been identified including 7q33 and isochromosome 1q. (Bhadra & Casey, 2006)

3. Embryology & genetics

Chordomas arise from remnants of the embryonic notochord and are located in all places where the notocord existed, including the clivus, sella turcica, foramen magnum, upper cervical spine and nasopharynx.

The notochord is a rod-like structure which comprises the embryonic axis of the body. It arises from ectodermal cells and forms during the third week of life. It is known to have an important role in the development of the vertebral column and is thought to play a part in somite differentiation, vertebral chondrogenesis and vertebral column segmentation as well as other possible roles. (Fleming et al, 2001)

During fetal life the notochord regresses but at the site of the intervertebral discs it persists and contributes to the formation of the nucleus pulposus. (Pazzaglia et al., 1989)

There is a large amount of evidence to support the theory that chordomas arise from notochordal cells. Portions of the notochord are known to persist at a number of sites including the skull base, coccyx and spine. These small, well-circumscribed, gelatinous collections of cells were first described by Muller, as ecchordoses physaliphoria. (Muller H, 1858) There is a morphological similarity between the cells of chordomas and ecchordoses physaliphoria. (Ribbert H, 1895) The immunohistological similarity between chordomas and notochord cells has been demonstrated in a number of studies. In addition, a study by Salisbury et al. (1993) demonstrated that although the notochord is a rod-like structure the rostral and caudal ends of the notochord are more complicated structures that demonstrate forking at the ends with fragments of chordal tissue separate from the main bulk of the notochord. This anatomical feature may help explain why regression of the notochord in fetal life may leave behind collections of notochordal cells which may subsequently give rise to chordomas in the common sites such as the skull base and sacrococcygeal region. (Salisbury et al., 1993)

Cytogenetic studies of chordoma show a number of abnormalities including triploidy, marker chromosomes, losses of or from chromosomes 1,3,4,10 and 13, and gains of chromosomes 7 and 20. (DeFrancesco et al., 2006) Microsatellite instability resulting from DNA mismatch repair deficiencies has also been demonstrated. (Klingler et al., 2000) However, no chordoma-specific translocations have yet been identified.

4. Pathology

Chordomas are typically found in three locations in the spine, with 50% occurring in the sacrum. The second most common site is the clivus, accounting for 35% of tumours and they are also seen less commonly in any part of the vertebral column. Other intraaxial and extraxial sites have been reported in the literature.

The site of origin of skull base chordomas is the clivus. From here they can extend into the anterior fossa, middle fossa, the sellar and parasellar regions and through the foramen magnum into the upper cervical spine. In the majority of cases the typical histological appearances and characteristic location of chordomas renders the diagnosis straightforward.

Chordomas are typically multilobulated masses. They are soft and gelatinous with a well-defined, greyish surface. The cut surface is usually homogenous but calcifications and occasional haemorrhages may be seen. However, chordomas are not histologially encapsulated and extensions of the fibrous tissue on the surface penetrate the tumour as fibrous septa creating a lobular appearance.

Microscopically chordomas are composed of relatively uniform populations of cells with cytoplasmic vacuoles of varying sizes. This abundant cell type is the pathognomic physaliphorous cells, while some cells have signet ring morphology and others have a more eosinophilic cytoplasm. The tumour cells are embedded in an basophilic and mucinous matrix. The cell nuclei are usually small, round or oval, with a dense chromatin pattern but occasional tumours may contain focal pleomorphism. Mitoses, although present, are usually rare. Mild atypia may be present but necrosis is uncommon. (Figure 1)

The cells of chordomas contain glycogen, and the matrix stains positively with mucicarmine and Alcian blue and metachromatically with toluidine blue. Ultrastructural examination of chordomas shows evidence of epithelial differentiation, with the presence of cell junctions and intracytoplasmic connections. Membrane-bound glycogen, intermediate filaments and rough endoplasmic reticululm are also found.

Chordomas stain positive for a number of immunohistochemial markers including positivity for cytokeratins, EMA, vimentin and occasionally S100 protein and carcinoembryonic antigen. Brachyury expression can also be used to distinguish them from other tumours such as chondrosarcoma. However, actin, demin, CD31, CD34 and collagen are usually negative. (DeFrancesco et al., 2006)

Variations of chordomas containing cartilaginous tissue have been described as chondroid chordomas. These account for a third of clival chordomas, have a slight female preponderance and occur in a younger age group. Those containing areas of sarcoma are described as dedifferentiated chordomas and they have a high risk of metastasis and a poor prognosis. The dedifferentiated component is usually not seen at presentation but occurs after recurrences and sometimes radiotherapy.

A few other lesions can mimic the appearance of chordoma on histology. These include chordoid meningioma, chondroma, chondrosarcoma (Figure 2), melanoma and metastatic adenocarcinoma. However, these lesions can usually be differentiated using further laboratory techniques.

5. Symptoms and signs

The craniovertebral region is a vital entry and exit point for a number of important neural pathways and structures. The precise nature of these clinical features and symptom progression depends entirely on the location of the chordoma and the rapidity of growth into the vital adjacent structures. It is therefore imperative that a thorough clinical history and clinical examination are undertaken to elucidate as much clinical information as possible at the time of diagnosis.

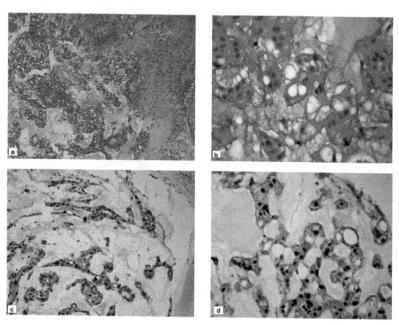

Fig. 1. a&b) H&E staining showing characteristic features of a chordoma (x40 & x100). Typical sheets of cells with cells containing vacuoles of various sizes can be seen. At higher magnification the phylasipharous cell, with it's large vaculole, can be easily made out as the abundant cell type. c&d) Brachyury immunohistochemistry identifying the characteristic chordoma cells.

Patients with chordomas at the CV junction can present in a number of ways including symptoms and signs of central and peripheral nervous system dysfunction. Clinical features can include sensory or motor disturbances, problems with gait, proprioception, coordination and respiratory compromise.

Neck pain is a presenting feature in 86% of patients. (Choi et al., 2010) Pain may occur in a dermatomal distribution, especially if the C2 nerve root is involved, but this is not always the case. Due to the propensity of chordomas to cause bone destruction the neck pain is usually non-specific and can sometimes be attributed to degenerative changes, particularly in older patients who do not have other features suggestive of more sinister disease at this location. Myelopathy is a common presenting feature, present in 18.6% of patients (Choi et al., 2010) and this may lead to weakness of the hands and associated spasticity of the extremities due to compression of the corticospinal tracts. (Crockard et al., 1993) Rarely a syrinx may be a present and these patients may present with atrophy of upper limb muscles and sensory disturbances.

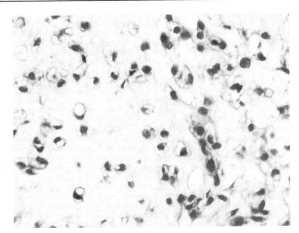

Fig. 2. H&E staining demonstrating chondrosarcoma (x100). The cells are not always arranged in a dense sheet like manner and contain less vacuoles and no phylasipharous cell. However, there are different grades of chondrosarcoma, which can all have slightly different appearances which need to be distinguished from chordoma using immunohistochemistry.

A number of cranial nerve deficits can result from chordomas at this location. Compression of the pons, medulla and rostral cervical region can lead to dysfunction of the trigeminal nucleus. In addition some branches of the facial, glossopharyngeal and vagus nerves supplying sensation to the face and tongue may also be affected as well as the motor supply to the palate. In addition, the accessory nerve may be compressed as it travels through the foramen magnum leading to motor deficits of the sternocleidomastoid and trapezius muscles. Chordomas located at the ventral surface of the foramen magnum may lead to compression of the hypoglossal nerve, which leads to ipsilateral tongue dysfunction and atrophy. If the jugular foramen is involved by the spread of chordoma then a number of distinct neurological syndromes may arise including Vernets, Collet-Sicard amd Villaret Syndromes. (Svien et al., 1969)

6. Imaging

Radiological diagnosis of CV junction chordomas has improved with advent of modern imaging modalities. Tumour location and extent of skull base involvement can now be precisely defined. Computed tomography (CT) and Magnetic Resonance Imaging (MRI) provide the mainstay of diagnostic information. However, plain radiographs, especially lateral radiographs of the cervical spine also have an important role to play, particularly in the postoperative assessment of cervical spine instrumentation. (Figures 3 a & b)

High resolution CT of the CV junction with bone and soft-tissue windows is very sensitive for detecting chordomas of the craniocervical junction. Fine cut axial and coronal unenhanced and contrast enhanced CT can evaluate bone involvement. On a CT scan, intracranial chordoma has a characteristic appearance with tumours being centrally located, well-defined, soft tissue masses arising from the clivus and causing lytic bone destruction. (Figure 4) Chordomas are usually hyper attenuating lesions and on administration of intravenous contrast they show a degree of enhancement.

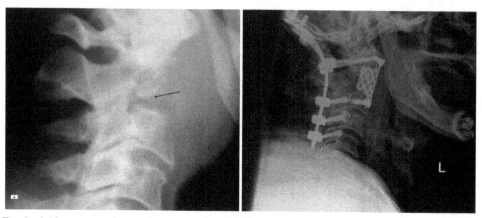

Fig. 3. a) Plain cervical spine lateral radiograph demonstrating osteolytic bone destruction in the region of the odontoid peg (arrow) . The chordoma mass can be seen anterior to the osteolyitc bone destruction, pushing the pharyngeal tissues anteriorly b) Post-operative plain cervical spine radiograph showing C2 corpectomy with insertion of cage and instrumented occipitocervical fusion using screws and rod fixation system.

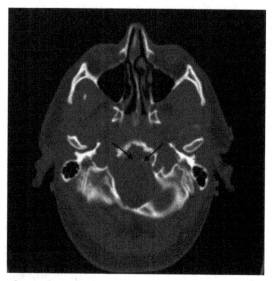

Fig. 4. Non-contrast enhanced axial CT of the craniovertebral junction, showing lytic bone destruction of the anterior clivus (arrows).

MRI of the CV junction is the best modality for evaluation of craniocervical junction chordomas. MR defines the extent of the tumour and it's spread to adjacent structures and is therefore useful both for diagnosis and for preoperative planning. Sagital images are the most useful as they define the posterior margin of the tumour and importantly, the relation to the brainstem and the nasopharyngeal extension of the chordoma. (Figures 5 a & b) Axial and coronal images are useful in detecting extension into surrounding structures.

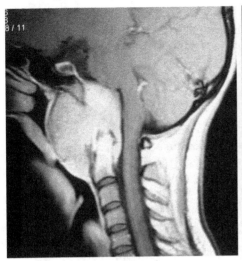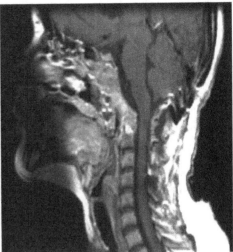

Fig. 5. a) Pre-operative T1 weighted sagital MRI showing extensive chordoma affecting the craniovetebral junction and spreading anteriorly to displace the pharyngeal structures. The tumour has a high signal and tumour expansion into the surrounding structures can be well delineated. b) Post-operative T1 weighted MRI of the craniovertebral junction showing resection of the tumour.

On T1 weighted MR imaging, chordomas usually demonstrate low signal intensity. Areas of high signal may be seen on T1 weighted images and these usually represent areas of focal haemorrhage. Chordomas classically have a high signal on T2-weighted MR scans due to their high fluid content. In addition T2 imaging is excellent for delineating the tumour from adjacent structures.

Craniovertebral junction chordomas demonstrate a degree of enhancement with gadolinium contrast. The enhancement is sometimes described as a 'honeycomb' appearance, which is due to intratumoural areas of low signal intensity. Fat suppression sequences can be used to differentiate tumour margins from adjacent fatty bone marrow. Small intraclival chordomas may be better demonstrated with these sequences.

MR Angiography (MRA) has a role in demonstrating the patency of the basilar artery as well as involvement of other large vessels including the internal carotid artery, which may be involved in large craniovertebral junction chordomas with significant anterior extension. Chordomas in this region often displace or encase vessels in this region and MRA has an advantage over digital subtraction angiography (DSA), which does not allow detection of encasement without luminal narrowing or occlusion. MRA is usually sufficient in pre-operative planning but DSA can demonstrate the collateral circulation and allow balloon occlusion of the internal carotid to help determine whether a patient is at risk if an important vessel is sacrificed.

Local recurrence of these tumours is a common finding and gadolinium enhanced MR is the best mode of assessing the degree of tumour excision and for follow-up. Marked high signal on T2 weighted imaging suggests tumour recurrence rather than post-operative changes.

The lesions most often confused with craniovertebral junction chordomas are chondroscarcomas. Although the majority of these usually occur in or around the sutures of the petrous bone, they can sometimes arise from the midline and mimic the MR appearance of a chordoma. Meningiomas arising from the clival region often do not cause bony destruction and tend to have a characteristic dural attachment.

6.1 Illustrative case

A 42-year-old man presented with a two-year history of neck pain, progressive difficulty in swallowing and visual disturbance. He had no significant medical problems and no family history of any illness. On examination he was alert and orientated in time, place and person. The only neurological deficit he had a left occulomotor and abducens nerve palsy. Plain radiographs of his cervical spine were unremarkable. Non-enhanced CT scan showed a lytic destruction of the anterior clivus (Figure 4). MR imaging was subsequently performed. The non-enhanced sagital T1-weighted MRI (Figure 5) demonstrated a large homogenous mass arising from the region of the craniovertebral junction and extending anteriorly compressing the pharyngeal structures. There is also associated lytic change within the odontoid peg. It was decided that the patient should have surgery to debulk the tumour followed by adjuvant radiation treatment. (See below)

7. Treatment

Harvey Cushing was the first surgeon to remove a chordoma successfully. (Cushing, 1912) Chordomas are usually extradural tumours that are found in the midline but they often extend into surrounding regions. There is a large body of evidence to suggest that maximal tumour resection is associated with a better outcome.

A number of approaches for the treatment of craniovertebral junction chordomas have been described but the most commonly used surgical approaches for lesions of the lower clivus, foramen magnum and the upper cervical spine is the standard transoral approach. A number of extended anterior midline transoral approaches exist including a transoral approach with a palatotomy, an 'open-door' maxillotomy, transmandibular and midface degloving procedures but the approach used depends on the exact site and extent of the lesion and surgeon experience and preference. More recently, endoscopic trans-nasal approaches have also been used with success.

All of the above approaches are suitable for midline clival chordomas but where there is significant lateral extension the midline approach alone may be insufficient for the removal of the entire tumour and more complex lateral approaches may have to be used as a primary or secondary procedure. A number of these approaches have been described for tumours of the upper clivus and include the subtemporal, transcavernous and the transpetrous approaches. (Gay et al., 1995a) For lateral lesions of the midclivus a subtemporal and infratemporal approach have been described. For lesions of the lower clivus with lateral extension to the occipital condyle and jugular foramen, the extreme lateral transcondylar approach can be used. (Sen & Sekhar, 1990) Larger chordomas involving the entire clival region, the sphenoid and the sellar region with extension anteriorly to the optic nerves may need staged surgery via multiple approaches.

7.1 Surgical approaches

The standard transoral approach is the main authors preferred approach to ventral midline craniocervical junction chordomas. It was first described by Kanavel (1908) who used it to remove a bullet between the skull base and atlas. This approach has since been modified and used to treat a number of aetiologies. (Kanavel, 1908) The standard transoral approach is the most frequently used approach for resecting chordomas of the craniocervical junction in the region of the lower clivus down to the level of C2. It may be combined with a soft palate split or an 'open-door' maxillotomy. Upper clival lesions may be excised using endoscopic trans-nasal techniques, which may have a lower complication rate than the 'open-door maxillotomy'.

Prior to performing the transoral procedure it is essential to ensure that the maximal interdental opening is greater than 25mm. A nasotracheal intubation is preferred and a nasogastric tube must be inserted. This ensures that the stomach is decompressed and more importantly, allows the administration of enteral nutrition following the procedure yet allowing the oropharyngeal wounds to heal. The patient's head is placed in a Mayfield head holder with the patient supine in the head-up position. The mouth is then cleaned with antiseptic solution, topical hydrocortisone applied to the mouth and oropharynx to reduce post-operative inflammation and parenteral antibiotics administered preoperatively and a further two doses following surgery.

The transoral retractor is inserted and the tongue blade ensures that the tongue is pushed down and out of the way. Insertion of the palatal retractors ensures that the palate is pulled upwards in the opposite direction and the nasotracheal and nasogastric tubes are pulled clear of the surgical field. The surgical anatomical landmark is the anterior tubercle of C1, to which is attached the anterior longitudinal ligament and the overlying longus colli muscle. A midline vertical incision is made on the tubercle of C1 and the pharyngeal retractors inserted and the longus colli muscle and the anterior longitudinal ligament cut using monopolar diathermy. This reveals the arch of C1 and the odontoid peg. The extent of the chordoma however, will dictate the craniocaudal and lateral extent of the exposure, and care should be taken to avoid damage to the hypoglossal nerve and the vertebral artery laterally. The C1 anterior arch and the peg are drilled out and the inferior clivus can be removed with drill and Kerisson rongeurs. The dural basilar plexus must be carefully dissected off the inferior border of the clivus to prevent vascular injury and bleeding. From here chordoma affecting the clivus can be resected. (Bouramas & Crockard, 2003)

If necessary the soft palate can be split in the midline to extend the superior and lateral exposure and this allows greater visualisation and access to the lower clivus. Another modification of the transoral procedure combines a LeFort I osteotomy with a midline incision in the hard and soft palate, the so-called 'open-door' maxillotomy. This provides excellent exposure to the upper middle clivus and sphenoid and gives good exposure inferiorly and laterally. For unilaterally extending tumours a unilateral LeFort osteotomy can be performed.

The endoscopic transnasal approach was developed to provide access to lesions of the middle and upper clivus and provides excellent visualization craniocervical junction. At the same time it avoids the complications of the traditional transoral approach and significantly reduces the morbidity associated with a LeFort osteotomy with 'open-door' maxillotomy. After the patient has undergone preoperative planning and the nasal anatomy has been assessed, the patient is put in a Mayfield head holder and topical adrenaline is applied to the nasal septum and mucosa of the turbinate bones. The entire procedure is performed under direct visualisation using an endoscope. The posterior aspect of the nasal septum is perforated near the rostrum of the sphenoid sinus to provide access to the nasopharynx. The rostrum of the sphenoid sinus is opened and the vomer and floor of the sphenoid sinus are removed. The mucosa of the nasophrynx is incised and usually reflected downwards into the oropaharynx and can be used as a flap at the end of the procedure. This allows visualisation of the anterior arch of C1 and the odontoid and resection of the tumour can then be performed. (Kassam et al., 2005)

Following an anterior approach to debulk the tumour a posterior occipito-cervical fixation is often required to provide stability to the upper cervical spine.

7.2 Surgical complications

A number of series have demonstrated high complication rates from excision of craniocervical junction chordomas. Harbour et al. (1991) reported 3 postoperative deaths in a series of 11 patients. Carpentier et al. (2002) reported 3 perioperative deaths in a series of 36 patients. Gay et al. (1995b) had a CSF leak rate of 30% and Pallini et al. (2003) reported 17 significant complications in 26 patients including 3 CSF fistulae. Choi et al. (2010) had a CSF leak rate of 6.2% and other complication rates included dysphagia (3.1%), nasal regurgitation (3.1%), meningitis (3.1%), sepsis (3.1%), chest infections, cranial nerve deficits and fixation failure. In the study by Choi et al. (2010), there were no differences in sepsis rates when comparing the standard transoral with the more extensive procedures. The study also showed that patients having the more extended surgeries appeared to have a worse prognosis than the standard transoral approach, although this was not statistically significant. It was also noted that patients who had their primary surgery at the specialist centres had a better outcome than those patients who had been initially treated elsewhere and had been referred on recurrence. Nasal regurgitation was more common with open-door maxillotomies than the standard procedure but the incidence of nasal regurgitation was not significantly different following division of the soft palate. Dysphagia was more common with mandibulotomy and glossotomy. (Choi et al., 2010)

It is clear that surgery confers a better survival benefit than with conservative treatment. Erikson et al. (1981) showed that survival rate for 11 patients with untreated chordoma was only 1 year. Radical resection of the tumour appears to confer the best survival outcomes as previously stipulated by Crockard et al. (2001) and also demonstrated by the large series of Choi et al. (2010). Colly & Al-Mefty (2001) achieved complete tumour excision in almost half of their patients with greater than ninety percent in almost 80%. However, they had a complication rate approaching 60%, with predominantly neurologic complications including cranial nerve palsies, cerebrospinal fluid leak, hydrocephalus, meningitis and oronasal fistulae. However, they found that complication rates did not greatly increase with greater extents of resection but there is a correlation of better survival with greater than 90% tumour resection. Gay et al. (1995) also demonstrated that there was no difference in complication rates in those patients receiving complete excision and those receiving partial debulking procedures. Although true oncological resection of these tumours is virtually impossible, aggressive tumour resection, including removal of bone margins where possible to reduce tumour load does appear to confer a survival benefit.

8. Radiation therapy

Despite the application of radiotherapy and radiosurgery for the treatment of CV junction chordomas, the importance of maximal surgical resection remains unequivocal. Greater survival has been shown to correlate with radical removal as opposed to partial resection. However, radical resection is not always possible due to the close proximity of these tumours to critical structures and the associated morbidity this entails. Traditionally chordomas have been regarded as relatively radio-resistant tumours but a number of treatment strategies using radiation treatments have been developed to gain control of these locally aggressive tumours. However, the size and precise location of the tumour is the most important factor in considering radiation planning.

Fractionated radiotherapy with high energy photons and radiotherapy with charged particles are the two most common forms of radiotherapy for CV junction chordomas. Fractionated radiotherapy has the benefit of sublethal damage repair of normal tissues in between treatment fractions, and thus the importance of surgery in resecting tumour from critical structures is vital.

8.1 Conventional radiation therapy

Conventional radiation therapy has been used for decades to gain local control of skull base chordomas and most patients undergo adjuvant fractionated radiotherapy to reduce the risk of tumour recurrence. However, initial doses of 50 to 55 Gy after resection did not provide successful local control and were associated with poor progression–free and overall survival rates. (Catton et al., 1996; Cummings et al., 1999) Catton et al reported on 13 patients who received a median dose of 50 Gy but only one of these patients remained disease free at 93 months following treatment. In the study by Cummings et al 24 patients diagnosed with chordoma were treated with megavoltage radiation therapy following incomplete tumour resection. The 5 year survival was 62% and at 10 years it was 28%.

Conventional radiotherapy with high energy photons, ranging from 40-70 Gy in different series, has been shown to be of survival benefit compared to surgery alone. However, local recurrence rates after residual incomplete resection followed by photon radiation therapy have been reported between 80% to 100%. (Catton et al., 1996; Cummings et al., 1999; Fuller & Bloom, 2003; Zorlu et al., 2000)

Although higher doses of fractionated radiotherapy have been shown to reduce the rate of tumour recurrence and increase survival rates, administration of higher doses are associated with greater side effects. Subsequently, other forms of radiation therapy have been pursued to greater success.

8.2 Proton beam radiation therapy

The largest amount of data in the use of radiation therapy for CV junction chordomas relates to proton beam therapy. Radiotherapy with charged particles has been used with success in the treatment of these tumours and has the advantage that it has a steeper fall-off then conventional therapy. Proton radiation allows improved dose localization than conventional photon therapy. In addition the positive charge of protons allows a energy dependent finite range in tissues, and the energy deposition demonstrates a sudden rise in dose at the end of the range with a subsequent sharp fall-off to zero dose, thereby providing excellent dose localization. This is known as the Bragg peak effect. Protons are assumed to have a slightly higher relative biological effectiveness compared with conventional photon radiotherapy. Proton beam radiation therapy is not restricted to the size of the tumour.

There are three large centres which have reported their outcomes of proton beam therapy in the literature: Loma Linda University Medical Centre (Loma Linda, CA), Harvard Cyclotron Laboratory at Massachusettes General Hospital (MGH/HCL) (Cambridge, MA) and the Institut Curie, Centre Protontherapie d'Orsay (Orsay Cedex, France)

The first patient to undergo proton irradiation for a CV junction chordoma was in 1974 at MGH/HCL. Since then, techniques have been developed to provide high dose, fractionated radiotherapy in doses excess of 70 Gy.

At LLUMC (Hug et al, 1999, 2001) Chordoma patients were treated with fractionated proton beam therapy to a mean dose of 70.7 CGE. The researchers observed a 3-year control rate of 67% with 5-year overall survival of 79%. In 1999 the MGN/HCL published there results of 519 cases of skull base tumours, of which 290 were chordomas. These patients were treated with combined proton and photon technique. The 5- and 10-year local recurrence free survival rates were 64% and 42% respectively. (Muzenrider & Liebsch, 1999) A hundred patients diagnosed with chordomas of the skull base and cervical spine were treated at the Centre de Protontherapie d'Orsay with a combined proton and photon technique. The median dose delivered to the tumour was 67 CGE. The 2- and 4-year local control rates were 86% and 54%.

Another form of charged particle therapy is the use of carbon ions, which also has a steep dose fall off after the Bragg peak. At the Gessellschaft fur Schwerionenforschung Darmstadt center in Heidelberg, Germany 96 patients with skull base chordoma were treated with carbon ion therapy. (Schulz-Ertner et al., 2007) The median dose delivered was 60 CGE with a mean follow-up time of 31 months. At 3 years, the local control rate in this series was 81% and 70% at 5-years. Overall survival rates were 92% and 89% at 3- and 5-years respectively.

The superior local tumour control and overall survival achieved using proton beam over conventional photon radiotherapy are due to the superior dose localisation characteristics of protons that result in a higher dose of radiation being delivered. However, side effects of this radiation therapy are relatively common and include the typical early and late radiation sequelae including nausea, headaches and radiation necrosis of the brain. It is important to note that there have not been any randomised trials comparing proton beam therapy to other types of radiation treatment.

8.3 Stereotactic radiosurgery

Stereotactic radiosurgery is a technique which is designed to achieve a greater radiobiological effect than conventional forms of radiotherapy. Due to its precision and steep dose fall off, stereotactic radiosurgery has been used as a minimally invasive primary, adjuvant and palliative management option in patients with CV junction chordomas.

Stereotactic radiosurgery is a potent treatment option for small sized chordomas. The greatest benefit of stereotactic radiosurgery is the steep dose gradient achievable, which minimizes radiation outside the tumour target, thus allowing the delivery of a larger dose to the tumour without exceeding the radiation-related tolerance of normal tissues.

The North American Gamma Knife Consortium (NAGKC) was established to evaluate the outcomes of patient with relatively rare tumours including chordomas. Their collaboration identified 71 patients who underwent stereotactic radiosurgery with Gamma Knife for chordoma. The median age of patients was 45 years and the median SRS target volume was 7.1 cm3 (range 0.9-109 cm3). Their study suggests that SRS is as effective as proton beam therapy for small tumours that have not been treated with prior radiation.

However, more rigorous studies need to be carried out to discover the relative merits of stereotactic radiosurgery over proton beam therapy.

For patients with craniocervical junction chordoma, maximal surgical resection with proton beam therapy remains the mainstay of treatment with stereotactic surgery possibly having a role in selected cases.

9. Medical therapies

Medical therapies do not routinely form the mainstay of treatment of chordomas. As with most other low grade malignancies these tumours are not reported to be sensitive to chemotherapy. A number of anecdotal reports of responses to chemotherapy exist (Azzarelli et al., 1988; McSweeney & Sholl, 1959; Razis et al., 1974; Scimeca et al., 1996) but these are limited to case reports. A prospective phase II clinical trial using the chemotherapy agent 9-nitro-camptothecin (9-NC), a topoisomerase inhibitor, has been conducted and although it only showed a 7% objective response rate it did demonstrate 6-month progression-free survival rate of 33% and a median time to progression of 9.9 weeks. (Chugh et al., 2005) No phase III clinical study of systemic therapy of chordomas been reported.

Other groups have attempted to investigate the effects of molecular targeted therapies as potential adjuvant treatments for low-grade chordomas. A phase II study of chordoma response to Imatinib Mesylate, a tyrosine kinase inhibitor, demonstrated a clinical benefit in 32 of 44 patients but reduction in tumour size was only observed in 7 of 44 patients. (Stacchiottis F et al., 2007)

In another study patients with PDGFR B positive inoperable or metastatic chordoma treated with imatinib mesylate, demonstrated stabilisation of the disease as a best response. (Ferraresi V et al., 2010) Other signal transduction pathways that may provide therapeutic targets include EGFR, which has been used in a single patient and showed clinical response. (Signal N et al., 2009)

Possible targets for immunotherapy include high molecular weight-melanoma associated antigen (HMW-MAA). This is expressed in over 60% of chordomas and studies have shown that this may be a useful target to apply immunotherapy to these tumours. (Schwab JH et al., 2009)

As laboratory and clinical investigations have started to reveal the genetic and molecular pathways involved in the pathogenesis of chordoma, future efforts may be focused on finding novel techniques to that can be translated into clinical practice.

10. Prognosis

Interpretation of published data on survival rates is difficult because of the heterogeneity of published series, small numbers of patients, short follow-up periods and difficulties in histological diagnoses, which has been common in earlier studies. Colli and Mefty (2001) documented a 5-year survival of 85.9% but this series included lesions, which may actually represent chondrosarcomas, which are known to have a better prognosis. In the large series by Choi et al 2010 the median survival rate was 84-months and the mean survival was 99 months from the date of surgery with 5- and 10-year survival times 55% and 36% respectively. Other studies have shown similar survival rates to this with Carpentier et al. (2002) having 5- and 10-year survival rates of 80% and 65% and Forsyth et al. (1993) showing survival rates of 51% and 35% following surgery.

11. Expert suggestions

Craniocervical junction chordomas are unique tumours that pose significant treatment challenges. As these lesions are rare we advocate that they should be treated at the first presentation at specialist centres where patients undergo careful selection and counselling and where specialists can perform a maximal resection of the tumour whilst keeping complications to a minimum.

12. Conclusion

Craniovertebral junction tumours are rare tumours that can present in a number of different ways. The majority of these tumours require radical surgery followed by adjuvant radiation therapy to improve outcome. Due to the heterogeneity of published series it is not possible to compare survival outcomes between existing series. However, due to the location of these tumours the prognosis remains poor.

13. Acknowledgements

The authors would like to thank the Dr Maria Thom, Consultant Neuropathologist at the National Hospital for Neurology and Neurosurgery, for supplying us with the histopathological images.

14. References

Azzarelli A, Quagliuolo V, Cerasoli S, Zucali R, Bignami P, Mazzaferro V, Dossena G & Gennari L. 1988. Chordoma: Natural history and treatment results in 33 cases. *Journal of Surgical Oncology*. 37(3):185-191.

Bhadra AK, Casey AT. 2006. Familial Chordoma. A report of two cases. *The Journal of Bone & Joint Surgery*. 88B:634-66.

Bouramas D & Crockard A. 2003. Anterior Odontoid Resection. In Surgical Techniques for the Spine. Haher TR, Merola AA. Pp 10-15. Thieme Medical Publishers, ISBN 3131247614, New York.

Carpentier A, Polivka M, Blanquet A, Lot G, George B. 2002. Suboccipital and cervical chordomas: The value of aggressive treatment at first presentation of the disease. *Journal of Neurosurgery*. 97:1070-1077.

Catton C, O'Sullivan B, Bell R, Laperriere N, Cummings B, Fornasier V & Wunder J. 1996. Chordoma: Long term follow-up after radical photon irradiation. *Radiotherapy & Oncology*. 41(1):67-72.

Chugh R, Dunn R, Zalupski MM, Bierman JS, Sondak VK, Mace JR, Leu KM, Chandler WF & Baker LH. 2005. Phase II study of 9-nitro-camptothecin in patients with advanced chordoma or soft tissue sarcoma. *Journal of Clinical Oncology.* 23(15):3597-604.

Choi D, Melcher R, Harms J, Crockard A. 2010. Outcome of 132 operations in 97 patients with chordomas of the craniocervical junction and upper cervical spine. *Neurosurgery.* 66(1):59-65.

Colli BO & Al-Mefty O. 2001. Chordomas of the skull base: follow-up review and prognostic factors. *Journal of Neurosurgery.* 95:933-943.

Crockard HA, Heilman AE, Stevens JM. 1993. Progressive myelopathy secondary to odontoid fractures: clinical, radiological and surgical features. *Journal of Neurosurgery.* 78(4)579-586.

Crockard HA, Steel T, Plowman N, Singh A, Crossman J, Revesz T, Holton JL, Cheeseman A. 2002. A multidisciplinary team approach to skull base chordomas. *Journal of Neurosurgery.* 95:175-183.

Cummings BJ, Hodson DI, Bush RS. 1999. Chordoma: The results of megavoltage therapy. *International Journal of Radiation Oncology, Biology, Physics.* 9:633-642.

Cushing H. 1912. The pituitary body and its disorders. Philadelphia: JB Lippincott.

DiFrancesco LM, Cristobal A, Castillo D, Temple WJ. 2006. Extra-Axial Chordoma. *Archives Pathological and Laboratory Medicine.* 130:1871-74.

Eriksson B, Gunterberg B, Kindblom LG. 1981. Chordoma: A clinicopathological and prognostic study of a Swedish national series. *Acta Orthopaedica Scandinavica.* 52:49-58.

Ferraresi V, Nuzzo C, Zoccali C, marandino F, Vidiri A, Salducca N, Zeuli M, Giannarelli D, Cognetti F, Biagini R. 2010. Chordoma: clinical characteristics, management and prognosis of a case series of 25 patients. *BMC Cancer.* 22:1471-2407.

Fleming A, Keynes RJ, Tannahill D. 2001. The role of the notochord in vertebral column formation. *Journal of Anatomy.* 199;177-80.

Forsyth PA, Cascino TL, Shaw EG, Scheithaeur BW, O'Fallon JR, Dozier JC, Piepgras DG. 1993. Intracranial chordomas: A clinicopathological and prognostic study of 51 cases. *Journal of Neurosurgery.* 78:741-747.

Fuller DB & Bloom JG. 2003. Radiotherapy for chordoma. *International Journal of Radiation Oncology, Biology, Physics.* 56:7-13.

Gay E, Sekhar LN, Wright DC. 1995a. Chordomas and chondrosarcomas of the cranial base. In Brain Tumours. Kaye AH, Laws ER Jr. Pp. 777-794. Churchill Livingstone, ISBN 0443048401, Edinburgh.

Gay E, Sekhar LN, Rubinstein E, Wright DC, Sen C, Janecka IP, Snyderman CH. 1995b.Chordomas and chondrosarcomas of the skull base: results and follow-up of 60 patients. *Neurosurgery.* 36:887-897.

Harbour JW, Lawton MT, Criscuolo GR, Holliday MJ, Mattox DE, Long DM. 1991. Clivus chordoma: A report of 12 recent cases and review of the literature. *Skull Base Surgery.* 1:200-206.

Kanavel AB. 1908. Bullet located between the atlas and the base of the skull: technique of removal through the mouth. *Surgical Clinics of Chicago.* 1:361-366.

Kassam AB, Gardner P, Snyderman C, Mintz A, Carrau R. 2005. Expanded endonasal approach: fully endoscopic, completely transnasal approach to the middle third of the clivus, petrous bone, middle cranial fossa and infratemporal fossa. *Neurosurgery Focus.* 15;19(1):E6.

Klingler L, Shooks J, Fiedler PN, Marney A, Butler MG. 2000. Microsatellite instability in sacral chordoma. *Journal of Surgical Oncology.* 73:100-3.

McSweeney AJ & Sholl PR. 1959. Metastatic chordoma use of mechlorethamine (nitrogen mustard) in chordoam therapy. *AMA Archives of Surgery.* 79:152-155.

Muzenrider JE & Liebsch NJ. 1999. Proton beam therapy for tumours of the skull base. *Strahlentherapie und Onkologie.* 175(Suppl 2):57-63.

Pallini R, Maira G, Pierconti F, Falchetti ML, Alvino E, Cimino-Reale G, Fernandez E, D'Ambrosio E, Larocca LM. 2003. Chordoma of the skull base: predictors of tumour recurrence. *Journal of Neurosurgery.* 98(4):812-822.

Pazzaglia UE, Salisbury JR, Byers PD. 1989. Development and involution of the notochord in the human spine. *Journal of the Royal Society of Medicine.* 82:413-415.

Muller H. 1858. Ueber das Vorkommen von resten der chorda dorsalis bei menschen nach der geburt und uber ihr verhaltniss zu den gallertgeschwulsten am clivus. *Z Ration Medic.* 2:202-229.

Razis DV, Tsatsaronis A, Kyriazides I et al. 1974. Chordoma of the cervical spine treated with vincristine sulfate. *Journal of Medicine.* 5:274-277.

Ribbert H. 1895. Uber die experimentelle Erzuegung einer Ecchondrosis physaliforia. *Verh Dtsch Kong Inn Med.* 13:455-464.

Rosenberg AE. 2003. Pathology of chordoma and chondrosarcoma of the axial skeleton. In: Chondromas and Chondrosarcomas of the Skull Base and Spine. Harsh GD, Janecka IP, Mankin HJ, Ojemann RG, Suit H, pp.8-15. Thieme Medical Publishers, ISBN 9783131247711, New York.

Salisbury JR, Deverell MH, Cookson JH & Whimster WF. 1993. Three dimensional reconstruction of human embryonic notochords: clue to the pathogenesis of chordoma. *Journal of Pathology.* 171:59-62.

Scimeca PG, James-Herry AG, Black KS, Kahn E & Weinblatt ME. 1996. Chemotherapeutic treatment of malignant chordoma in children. *Journal of Pediatric Hematology & Oncology.* 18:237-240.

Scwab JH, Boland PJ, Agaram NP, Socci ND, Guo T et al. 2009. Chordoma and chondrosarcoma gene profile: implications for immunotherapy. *Cancer Immunology & Immunotherapy.* 58:339-349.

Sculz-Ertner D, Karger CP, Feuerhake A, Nikoghosyan A, Combs SE, Jakel O, Elder L, Scholz M & Debus J. 2007. Effectiveness of carbon ion therapy in the treatment of skull base chordomas. *International Journal of Radiation Oncology, Biology, Physics.* 68:449-457.

Sen CS, Sekhar LN. 1990. An extreme lateral approach to intradural lesions of the cervical spine and foramen magnum. *Neurosurgery.* 27:197-204.

Singhal N, Kotasek D, Parnis FX. 2009. Response to erlotinib in a patient with treatment refractory chordoma. *Anticancer Drugs.* 20:953-955.

Stacchiottis FV, Ferraresi G, Grignani F, Crippa A, Messina E, Tamborini CS, Gronchi A, Casali PG. 2007. Imatinib mesylate in advanced chordoma: a multicenter phase II study. *Journal of Clinical Oncology.* 25:1000-1003.

Svien HJ, Baker HL, Rivers MH. 1969. Jugular foramen syndrome and allied syndromes. *Neurology.* 13:797-809.

Zorlu F, Gurkaynak M, Yildiz F, Oge K & Atahan IL. 2000. Conventional external radiotherapy in the management of clival chordomas with overt residual disease. *Neurological Science.* 21:203-207.

2

Balloon-Kyphoplasty for Vertebral Compression Fractures

Luca Arpino and Pierpaolo Nina

Department of Neurosurgery, San Giovanni Bosco Hospital, Naples
Italy

1. Introduction

1.1 Overview

A Vertebral Compression Fracture (VCF) is a collapse of one or more vertebrae. This usually results from a combination of bending forward and downward pressure on the spine. These fractures happen most commonly in the thoraco-lumbar spine, particularly in the lower vertebrae of the thoracic spine.

1.2 Causes

In relation to etiopathogenesis, VCFs may be divided into:

- pathologic fractures, as for:
  - *osteoporosis* (the most common cause: about 750,000 people per year in United States): in people with severe osteoporosis, a VCF may be caused by simple daily activities, such as stepping out of the shower, sneezing vigorously or lifting a light object;
  - *metastatic tumors;*
  - *multiple myeloma;*
  - *vertebral hemangiomas;*
- traumatic fractures, which can occur with a fall on the feet or buttocks, a forceful jump, a car accident or any event that stresses the spine past its breaking point.

1.3 Symptoms

VCFs may occur suddenly, causing severe back pain, generally referred to mid or lower part of the spine; this pain is most commonly described as "knifelike" and usually disabling. Clinical examination usually shows tenderness to the touch over the affected vertebra/vertebrae.

If the VCF is severe, the nerves and spinal cord can be affected, which can lead to nerve irritation and inflammation.

1.4 Imaging

While a diagnosis can usually be made through history and a clinical examination, X-ray and CT-scan (as first-step diagnosis in Emergency Room) or MRI and bone densitometry can help in confirming diagnosis, predicting prognosis, and determining the best treatment option for this patient.

1.5 Balloon-kyphoplasty (BKP) technique

BKP is a percutaneous vertebral augmentation technique initially developed to treat osteoporotic VCFs. It is a minimally invasive procedure: a small incision is made in the back through which the surgeon places a hollow tube called *trocar*. Using fluoroscopy to guide it to the correct position, the trocar creates a path into the fractured area through the pedicle of the involved vertebrae (*fig1*):

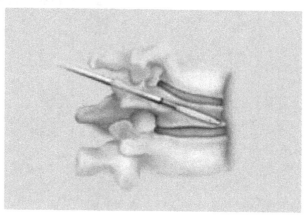

Fig. 1. Trocar insertion

Then a special balloon is inserted through the trocar into the vertebra and it is gently inflated by the surgeon (*fig2*):

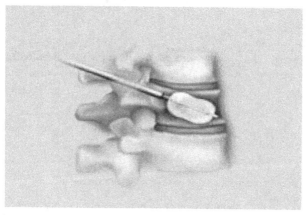

Fig. 2. Balloon inflation

As the balloon inflates, fractured vertebra is elevated while its inner cortical bone is compacted: so a cavity into the vertebra is created (*fig3*):

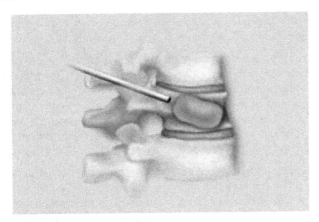

Fig. 3. Void filling by bone cement

Finally, the balloon is removed and the surgeon fills the cavity with bone cement in order to achieve fracture stabilization and body height restoration (*fig4*):

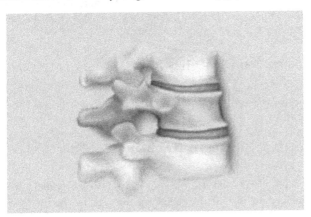

Fig. 4. Fracture stabilization

2. Alternative procedures

According to kind of VCF, related symptoms and health conditions, there are many ways to treat these fractures.

When permitted by a doctor, self-care at home, taking rest, with a back brace and/or using medications (nonsteroidal anti-inflammatories, narcotics or muscle relaxants) may be enough in case where pain is not so severe, neurological examination is negative and radiological tests show minor VCF.

On the other hand, admission to the hospital is necessary when pain or symptoms are severe. Surgery (major or mini-invasive spinal surgery depending on VCF degree) may be required to prevent the spine from pressing on the spinal cord or to stabilize the vertebra adjacent to the fracture site. When spinal cord compression is not a risk and neurological examination is negative instead, percutaneous techniques such as vertebroplasty or *vertebral augmentation techniques* such as BKP or stentoplasty are enough.

Unlike BKP, in **vertebroplasty** bone cement is injected into the vertebra at high pressure and *free*: so cement-leakage rate is higher, especially if there are many fracture cracks, such as for traumatic VCFs [Schmelzer et al, 2009]. In his meta-analysis on 69 clinical studies, Hulme [Hulme et al, 2006] reported leakage rates in 41% of cases during vertebroplasty and in 9% of cases during BKP. While most leaks were clinically asymptomatic, clinical complications (i.e. major complications) occurred in 3.9% and 2.2% of the vertebroplasty and kyphoplasty cases, of which pulmonary emboli accounted for 0.6% and 0.01%, respectively.

Vertebral body stenting (VBS), also known as **stentoplasty,** is a further adaptation of vertebroplasty and BKP. It is a new technique, recently developed, that involves placing a metal stent (cage) within the collapsed vertebral body and then expanding this to try and enable some height restoration before filling that cavity created with cement. The main advantage of VBS over BKP is that the height gain after balloon inflation can be maintained whereas with BKP alone it is well-known that in many cases significant height loss occurs during balloon deflation. However, after this procedure, stent remains into the vertebral body to keep vertebral body height restoration; furthermore the stent does not represent a *closed system* like the balloon: so cement-leakage rate is most likely higher than BKP, even though there are not longer follow-up studies for VBS.

3. Indications and contraindications of BKP

BKP is a broadly used method for the management of VCFs [Molina et al, 2011]. Originally introduced for osteoporotic fractures, surgical indications for this percutaneous vertebral augmentation technique were extended to vertebral fractures resulting from multiple myeloma [Zou et al, 2010], spinal metastases [Dalbayrak et al, 2010], vertebral hemangiomas [Jones et al, 2009] and trauma [Doria et al, 2010; Costa et al, 2009; de Falco et al, 2005].

In a recent study, Rollinghof et al. [Rollinghof et al, 2010] reported on a multiple choice questionnaire submitted to 580 clinics registered to practice BKP in Germany. For most participante (95,4% of the users), the main clinical indication was permanent back pain at the fractured level with an average VAS of 5. Although there is no common agreement about the etiopathogenetic and neuroradiological types of VCF to treat with kyphoplasty [Movrin et al, 2010, Bula et al, 2010, Dashti et al, 2005], over 80% of the users regarded A1.1, A1.2, and A3.1 fractures as main indications for kyphoplasty while for more than 60%, osteoporotic A1.1 fracture constituted the main indication for vertebroplasty [Rollinghof et al, 2010]. Although gradual pain resolution following these fractures is the expected natural history, pain can persist and or resolve slowly with conservative management. While patients may be not responsive to non-surgical therapies [Nairn et al, 2011]. Furthermore – especially in osteoporotic patients – VCFs can be complicated by deformity, loss of stature, impairment of pulmonary function and (considering that most VCFs will heal in 8 - 10 weeks with rest, bracing, and pain medications[Klazen et al, 2010]) the attendant risks of poor mobility/immobilisation in the elderly, such as venous thrombo-embolism or discomfort. Whereas BKP could allow rapid pain relief, as well as improved physical function and quality of life [Ledlie et al, 2006].

Obvious contrainticatons to BKP are pregnancy, congenital or aquired coagulopathies (warfarin, ASA), pain unrelated to vertebral collapse, fractured pedicles, solid tumors, osteomyelitis, contrast allergy (balloons are filled with contrast that can extravasate if they rupture), complete loss of vertebral height (vertebra plana).

4. Preoperative planning

A plain X-ray of the spine is generally enough to make the radiographic diagnosis of VCF (fig5):

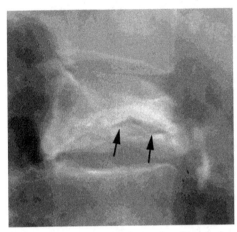

Fig. 5. 71-year-old woman with traumatic VCF. Lateral radiographs of lumbar spine show loss of vertebral body height and linear well-demarcated radiolucency characteristic of intravertebral fracture cleft (arrows).

CT is the most sensitive means to evaluate the location, severity, and extension of the collapsed vertebra, as well as to ascertain the visibility of the vertebral pedicles and the integrity of the posterior wall [Masala et al, 2004] (fig6):

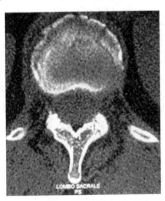

Fig. 6. 52-year-old woman with traumatic VCF of L1. Axial CT scan showing Magerl A1.2 type fracture of the vertebra.

Furthermore, CT scan of the spine allows multi-planar reconstructions, very useful to classify a traumatic VCF according to AO-Magerl classification (*fig7-8*) [Magerl et al, 1994]:

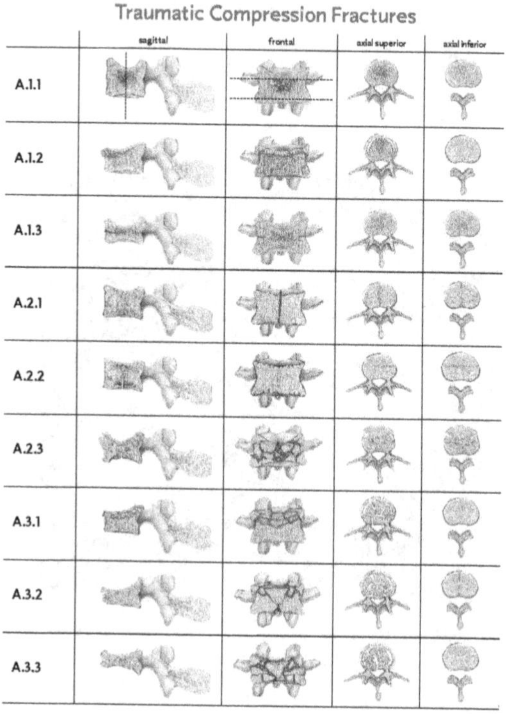

Traumatic Compression Fractures

	sagittal	frontal	axial superior	axial inferior
A.1.1				
A.1.2				
A.1.3				
A.2.1				
A.2.2				
A.2.3				
A.3.1				
A.3.2				
A.3.3				

Fig. 7. AO-Magerl classification for type-A fractures

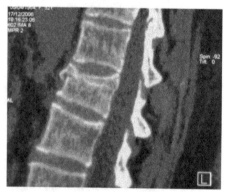

Fig. 8. 52-year-old woman with traumatic VCF of L1. Sagittal CT reconstruction of the previous fracture.

MRI is essential in identifying cord compression as consequence of a posteriorly displaced bone fragment, especially at levels where spinal cord is present (e.g. from the cervical spine to second lumbar vertebra) (*fig9*):

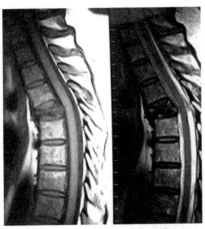

Fig. 9. 49-year-old woman with pathologic (myeloma) VCF. Sagittal MRI of the spine showing mild cord compression at T6 level by a displaced bone fragment.

When there is no data about the timing of fracture, it is important to perform a specific sequence MRI (e.g. STIR, *Short Tau Inversion Recovery*) scan before a kyphoplasty or vertebroplasty procedure is carried out, since it is impossible to distinguish between an old, healed fracture and a new fracture on X-rays or a CT scan. STIR MRI, in fact, is an inversion recovery pulse sequence with specific timing so as to suppress the signal from fat; in this way, the focal hyperintensity (bone marrow edema) that lasts for 2-4 months after fracture can be distinguished from fat signal, suggesting an acute or subacute VCF [Masala et al, 2004].

Finally, bone scintigraphy is helpful in assessing metastatic disease and when pain is elicited on palpation at levels other than where a fracture is radiographically identified (*fig10*):

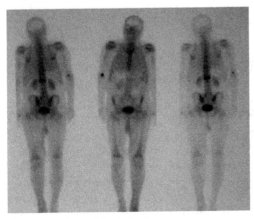

Fig. 10. Bone scan showing an acute vertebral fracture.

5. Key steps of the procedure

As is done in many surgical procedures, prophylactic antibiotics are administered to the patient approximately 30 minutes before the actual procedure; however, the efficacy of this practice in preventing infection has never been affirmed by controlled study [Mathis et al, 2001].

BKP is usually not painful and requires only intravenous mild sedation and local anesthesia. The local anesthetic is injected in to the skin, subcutaneous tissues, and periosteum of the vertebra. General anesthesia is another possible choice, especially for lengthy cases involving numerous levels of vertebral fractures; but local anesthesia with sedation is generally enough, especially when general anesthesia is contraindicated by patient's health conditions (e.g. pathologic VCFs in tumors, myeloma, etc.) [Lavelle et al, 2007].

Prone positioning is achieved and a C-arm is provided; biplane fluoroscopy will allow simultaneous visualization in two projections during injection of bone cement. It allows the procedure to be performed more rapidly [Wehrli et al, 1995] and is often chosen when the procedure is performed in a radiology department because of equipment availability and familiarity.

After fluoroscopic localization, a small incision is made and a thin cannulated trocar with bone biopsy needle is advanced to the antero-posterior radiographic projection of the pedicle. Then the cannula is passed through the pedicle into the vertebral body being treated. Both lateral and antero-posterior projections provide necessary visualization of the path of the needle. An alternative approach is the extrapedicular. This is most often used to access the upper thoracic spine, where pedicles are smaller then in the lumbar tract. The extrapedicular approach involves inserting the cannula between the lateral margin of the pedicle of thoracic vertebrae and the rib head [Hide et al, 2004]. When fracture fragments are reached, the needle is removed and a drill bit is inserted into the cannula; so a passage to the anterior part of the vertebral body is created. Then a void is created within the cancellous bone by an inflatable bone tamp prior to cement delivery (*fig1 and 2*): in this way, bone cement is not *free*, cement-leakage rate is considerably lower than vertebroplasty and a lower pressure is needed to inject bone cement into the vertebra (*fig3*). Occasionally patients report pain when a tool is removed too quickly from the cannula, reasonably due to the sudden negative pressure. This procedure takes about one hour or less for each vertebra involved.

Sometimes kyphoplasty allows achieving height restoration of the fractured vertebral body, thus preventing kyphosis – therefore *kyphoplasty* (*fig4*).

6. Postoperative care

Recovery from a kyphoplasty is relatively quick. In our experience, patients feel almost immediate pain relief after the surgery. Most patients can go home on the day of the procedure; however we prefer to discharge the patient the day after, so he/she may obtain adequate information from our staff about post operative care at home. During hospitalization, in fact, the nurse staff will provide the patient with medication for pain and will encourage him/her to get up, and move around, as soon as possible after the surgery. Bending or sitting should be avoided for an hour or more. Most patients are very satisfied with the procedure and are able to gradually resume activity once discharged from the hospital. Once at home, patients may resume their activities of daily living as soon as they are able. The bandages may be removed two or three days after they return home from the hospital; the incision on the back should require very little care: keeping it clean and dry is the best. Showering is allowed after only one day, but the patient should not take a bath or go swimming for three weeks. Driving or lifting of heavy objects is forbidden until after about two weeks.

Postoperative bracing is unnecessary, because bone cement hardens during the procedure (PMMA) or within one hour after it (CPC): in fact, the resistance to compressive forces of CPC has been demonstrated not to differ significantly from PMMA after in vitro vertebroplasty in human cadavers [Bai et al, 1999] while another in vitro study reported that CPC can attain compressive strength comparable to that of an intact vertebral body within 15-20 minutes after implantation: thus, the biomaterial is sufficiently strong for safe transfer of the patient within a reasonable time, following setting (bed-rest for 24h after BKP with CPC is suggested by this study: that's what we do) [Schwardt et al, 2006].

An appointment for radiological and clinical follow-up is scheduled a month after discharge: patients will come to hospital with a plain X-ray of the spine and blood tests (looking for indicators of an acute phase response).

7. Complications

The most commonly described complication is an extravertebral leakage of bone cement [Groen et al, 2004], more likely in traumatic VCFs compared to pathologic VCFs due to more fracture cracks in traumatic fracture [Schmelzer-Schmied et al, 2009]. The systematic review of the literature by Hulme found rates of cement leakage in vertebroplasty of 41% (n = 2283 levels) and in kyphoplasty of 9% (n = 1486 levels) of treated vertebrae. This can lead to spinal stenosis or to pulmonary cement embolism [Choe et al, 2004]. But most leaks were clinically asymptomatic: consider that leaks-distribution is mainly paraspinal (48%) and intradiscal (38%), then epidural (11%) and finally pulmonary (1.5%) and foraminal (1.5%) [Hulme et al, 2009]. In our series, there is a 33% of asymptomatic cement-leakage rate.

In addition, systemic allergic or toxic reactions to bone cement have been described [Kalteis et al, 2004]. New fractures of adjacent vertebrae occurred for both procedures at rates that are higher than the general osteoporotic population but approximately equivalent to the general osteoporotic population that had a previous vertebral fracture [Hulme et al, 2009].

8. Clinical series and outcome

In his systematic review of 69 clinical studies, Hulme compared outcomes from vertebroplasty and kyphoplasty [Hulme et al, 2009]: in both case a large proportion of subjects had some pain relief independent of the type of procedure (87% vertebroplasty, 92% kyphoplasty). Visual analog pain scores (VAS) (normalized to 10-point scale) were reduced from an average of 7.15 to 3.4 for BKP while only two kyphoplasty studies reported on improvement in physical function [Ghros et al, 2006; Gaitains et al, 2005]: this suggests that reporting improvements in physical function appears to be of secondary importance to the investigators; therefore, measurement scales used are inconsistent and scores cannot be pooled [Hulme et al, 2009]. The pain relief experienced by patients appears to be promising for both BKP and vertebroplasty in the short-term (<1 year) whereas it appears that pain relief is durable: in fact, little change was noted between postoperative scores and long-term. [Hulme et al, 2009, Zoarski et al, 2002]. However, note that long-term follow-up results were not as frequently reported [Hulme et al, 2009]

A qualitative examination of the data collected by Hulme indicates that vertebral height restoration is similar both for vertebroplasty and BKP (mean 6.6°). However, interstudy comparisons are further complicated by the use of different methods for percentage height restoration and reduction of kyphosis angle calculation [Hulme et al, 2009, McKiernan et al, 2003]. As described in the section above, cement leaks occurred for 41% and 9% of treated vertebrae for vertebroplasty and kyphoplasty respectively, while adjacent level fracture rates are similar between both procedures and approximately equivalent to the general osteoporotic population that had a previous vertebral fracture. Furthermore, the stabilization of a specific fracture level by kyphoplasty may lead to secondary fractures of adjacent vertebrae due to the changed biomechanics of the spine [Baroud et al, 2006, Berlemann et al, 2002]. However, these studies refer to osteoporotic VCFs, so the adjacent vertebral fractures are related to a low bone density [Tseng et al, 2009].

8.1 Our series

From March 2005 to March 2011, 137 hospitalized patients underwent BKP for VCF at our Department. Among these, 76 patients (55,5%) fulfilled the criteria set at our Institution to be offered BKP after having suffered traumatic VCF (tab1):

Parameters		N = 76
Gender (M)		40 (52.6%)
Level (>=2)		2 (2.6%)
Magerl		
	A 1.2	31 (43.0%)
	A 1.3	14 (19.4%)
	A 3.1	27 (37.5%)
Age		53±15
VAS pre		8.8±1.1
VAS post		3.0±2.0
DeltaVAS		67±21

Table 1. Demographic and clinical charatteristics; DeltaVAS = (VAS pre-VAS post)/VAS pre)*100

Inclusion criteria were:

1. no neurological deficits;
2. one or, at most, two vertebral body injuries involving the spine from T5 through L4 or, when feasible, L5;
3. no radiological evidence of mechanical instability;
4. Magerl nonsurgical and stable fractures, that are – in our opinion – A1.2 (wedge impaction) (N=31), A1.3 (vertebral body collapse) (N=14) and A3.1 (incomplete burst

fracture) types without retro-pulsed fragment. We exclude A2.1 to A2.3 types because there is always a split of the vertebral body that could allow cement leakage.

Mean age was 53±15 years and 53% males. Mean preoperative VAS was 8.7±1.1 while Postoperative VAS was 3.0±2.0 significantly lower with p-value<0.0001. As reported in *graph1*:

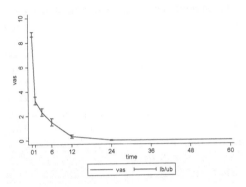

Graph. 1. Outcome: pain-relief during follow-ups; lb = lower bund, ub = upper bund

VAS decreased significantly after surgery while complete pain releif was obtained at 2-year follow-up for 42 patients; this result is durable for 8 patients with 6-year follow-up. We believe that, unlike patients with pathologic VCFs, in traumatic patients healthy conditions are good (no osteoporosis, tumors or myeloma): so a complete pain relief is a possible goal after BKP.

Early mobilization (i.e., within 24-48h from BKP) was obtained in all cases. Because our philosophy is to not overfill traumatic fractured vertebra, height restoration is not our target for this kind of VCFs. So we didn't take any measurement of Cobb angle. In 23 subjects (30%) asymptomatic cement leakages occurred.

9. Traumatic VCFs: Tips and tricks

Because we work closely with our Emergency Department, more than 50% of our cases are traumatic VCFs

One of the most controversial issues millitating against BKP in traumatic VCFs relates to the main bone cement used in this procedure (i.e. poly-methlyl-metacrylate, PMMA), which cannot integrate into bone and can not allow for bone-healing.

On the contrary, we prefer to use PMMA because the potential local reaction to PMMA (incidental to the exothermic reaction that occurs while the PMMA bone cement is hardening *in situ*) brings fibrous tissue formation at the interface between bone and bone cement [Kalteis et al, 2004], which may be a serious disadvantage for a joint (e.g. hip) but seems not to be significant for a non-articulating bone such as the vertebral body.

However, we suggest some care in performing BKP in traumatic VCF:

1. In traumatic factures there is much higher rate of cement leakage compared to non-traumatic VCF; this is due to the nature of these traumatic fractures: the cement can leak

through the many fracture cracks [Schmezler-Schmied et al, 2009]. So we prefer to not overfill the fractured vertebra with cement because an excessive amount of bone cement could lead to a higher rate of leakage. This also explains why we mainly prefer kyphoplasty over vertebroplasty, which needs a much higher pressure.

2.   Unlike osteoporotic VCFs, it's very difficult to achieve height restoration in traumatic fractures because these patients have a normal bone density [Schmezler-Schmied et al, 2009]: so over-inflating the balloon seems to be unnecessary. Higher rates of cement leakage and/or balloon burst are present.

3.   Because a low risk of adjacent vertebral fractures is described for vertebral augmentation techniques (generally for vertebroplasty) with PMMA cement [Gerztbein et al, 1994; Kalteis et al, 2004; Tseng et al, 2009], we prefer to not overfill the fractured vertebra keeping this risk to the minimum: reported clinical studies have shown that even "insufficient" filling of vertebral bodies during a vertebroplasty can lead to a successful outcomes in pain reduction, and stiffening and stabilizing of the fractured vertebrae [Luo et al, 2007; Furtado et al, 2007; Oakland et al, 2009]. The mechanism for adjacent vertebral fractures is still unclear, but from experimental and computational studies, it appears that vertebroplasty changes the mechanical loading in adjacent vertebrae because of excessive cement rigidity of treated vertebra [Baroud et al, 2006; Berlemann et al, 2002]. However, it is noted that these studies refer to VCF from osteoporosis, so the adjacent vertebral fractures are related to a low bone density. In fact, Tseng concluded that older patient ages, lower baseline BMD, and more pre-existing vertebral fractures were found to be risk factors for multiple vertebral compression fractures [Tseng et al, 2009].

4.   Inflammatory response to PMMA exothermic reaction could lead to bone resorption all around this cement. Although this is a serious disadvantage for prostheses integration into the bone (a common technique to aid in implant fixation into surrounding bone is to inject bone cement into the space between the implant and surrounding bone [Kuhn et al, 2000]), this seems not to be very significant for a non-articulating bone, as represented by a vertebral body, especially if we consider that some authors successful treated intravertebral pseudarthroses (whose neuroradiological findings is are the rare and, so-called, *intravertebral vacuum fenomenon* [Van Eenenaan et al, 1993]) by BKP with PMMA [Ghros et al, 2006]. Furthermore, Aebli has shown that temperature levels after usage of intravertebral PMMA cement may be sufficient to cause intravertebral thermal necrosis, but that heat levels outside the vertebral body (e.g. at the intervertebral discs and vertebral endplates) are unlikely to cause thermal injury [Aebli et al, 2006]. However, we prefer to keep to a minimum the amount of cement in order to avoid local bone resorption.

5.   Finally, we agree with de Falco [de Falco et al, 2005] about the opportunity to use bioactive cement in patients under 50 years. In fact, although the use of PMMA cement in vertebroplasty is widespread, no data on the long-term behaviour of the material for spinal applications has been published. So, because the majority of patients with traumatic vertebral fractures are aged less than 50 years and the PMMA material remains inside the vertebral body for life, the use of more biocompatible bone cement is preferred [Verlaan et al, 2002]. Thus, the usage of calcium phosphate cement (CPC), which hardens by crystallization at body temperature, avoids thermal injury, whereby it is unclear whether thermal necrosis actually contributes to the fibrous tissue layer around PMMA implants [Libicher et al, 2006]. However, we have to take into

consideration the fact that bioactive cements are much more expensive than PMMA. Therefore, it may be that the use of very expensive bone cement is deemed innaproriate for elderly patients.

10. Explicative cases

We present two illustrative cases about among our procedures.

10.1 Case 1

52-year-old female, L1 traumatic A1.2 vertebral compression fracture (*fig. 11*):

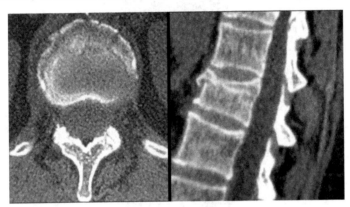

Fig. 11. Case 1. Axial (right) and sagittal MPR (left) CT scan of L1 traumatic A1.2 VCF. Posterior vertebral wall is untouched.

As you can see in the postoperative CT scan (*fig. 12*):

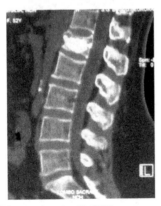

Fig. 12. Case 1. Postoperative CT scan (sagittal MPR)

L1 body was not overfilled by bone cement (PMMA), because our target for traumatic VCFs is stabilization *not* augmentation. X-ray follow-up at 2 (*fig. 13*) and 5 years (*fig. 14*) are showed:

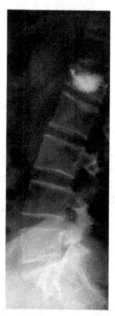

Fig. 13. Case 1. X-ray follow-up (2 years)

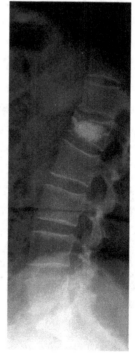

Fig. 14. Case 1. X-ray follow-up (5 years)

Stabilization was held, no further collapse of the kyphoplastied vertebra or adjacent fractures were seen at long-term follow-up. Preoperative VAS was 7 while postoperative VAS became 0 since three months after BKP; this clinical goal was kept at 5 years follow-up.

10.2 Case 2

This is one of first case of our series. 53-year-old male, T12 traumatic A3.1 vertebral compression fracture (*fig. 15*):

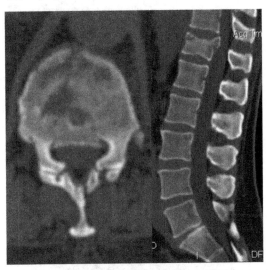

Fig. 15. Case 2. Axial (right) and sagittal MPR (left) CT scan of T12 traumatic A3.1 VCF. Intact pedicles are clearly visible in axial scan. Non-significant retropulsed fragment is present.

As you can see in post-operative CT-scan (fig16):

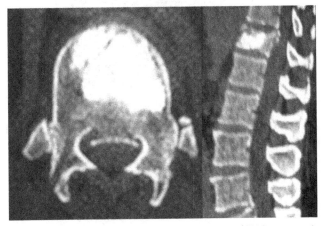

Fig. 16. Case 2. Axial (right) and sagittal MPR (left) CT scan of D12 traumatic A3.1 VCF after BKP. Vertebral body was not overfilled while retropulsed fragment wasn't touched.

we used a little amount of bone cement to fill the vertebral body: stabilization was achieved while vertebral body augmentation was poor; this "undercharging" philosophy was also useful in not touching the retropulsed fragment.

This radiographic result was held after 6-years follow-up (fig17):

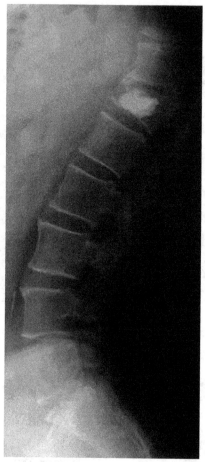

Fig. 17. Case 2. X-ray follow-up (6 years)

Pre-operative VAS was 8 while post-operative VAS significantly improved to 2; complete absence of pain was achieved 6 months after BKP, and this score was held at 6-years follow-up-

11. Conclusion

In our experience, BKP is a safe and effective procedure to treat nonsurgical and stable traumatic VCF compared to conservative therapy and to other percutaneous augmentation technique such as vertebroplasty.

Although long-term studies about effectiveness of BKP for traumatic VCFs are unsatisfactory, our 6-years follow-up suggests that this vertebral-augmentation technique represent a very attractive, easy and fully adequate solution to treat this kind of traumatic fractures.

12. Acknowledgments

Special thanks to Chris Johnson for correcting English usage in my paper

13. References

Aebli N, Goss BG, Thorpe P, Williams R, Krebs J. In vivo temperature profile of intervertebral discs and vertebral endplates during vertebroplasty: an experimental study in sheep. Spine (Phila Pa 1976). 2006 Jul 1;31(15):1674-8; discussion 1679.

Bai B, Jazrawi LM, Kummer FJ, Spivak JM. The use of an injectable, biodegradable calcium phosphate bone substitute for the prophylactic augmentation of osteoporotic vertebrae and the management of vertebral compression fractures. Spine (Phila Pa 1976). 1999 Aug 1;24(15):1521-6.

Baroud G, Vant C, Wilcox R. Long-term effects of vertebroplasty: adjacent vertebral fractures. J Long Term Eff Med Implants. 2006;16(4):265-80.

Berlemann U, Ferguson SJ, Nolte LP, Heini PF. Adjacent vertebral failure after vertebroplasty. A biomechanical investigation. J Bone Joint Surg Br. 2002 Jul;84(5):748-52.

Bula P, Lein T, Straßberger C, Bonnaire F. Balloon Kyphoplasty in the Treatment of Osteoporotic Vertebral Fractures: Indications - Treatment Strategy - Complications. Z Orthop Unfall. 2010 Nov 15. [Epub ahead of print]

Choe DH, Marom EM, Ahrar K, Truong MT, Madewell JE. Pulmonary embolism of polymethyl methacrylate during percutaneous vertebroplasty and kyphoplasty. AJR Am J Roentgenol. 2004 Oct;183(4):1097-102.

Costa F, Ortolina A, Cardia A, Sassi M, De Santis A, Borroni M, Savoia G, Fornari M. Efficacy of treatment with percutaneous vertebroplasty and kyphoplasty for traumatic fracture of thoracolumbar junction. J Neurosurg Sci. 2009 Mar;53(1):13-7.

Costa F, Ortolina A, Cardia A, Sassi M, De Santis A, Borroni M, Savoia G, Fornari M. Efficacy of treatment with percutaneous vertebroplasty and kyphoplasty for traumatic fracture of thoracolumbar junction. J Neurosurg Sci. 2009 Mar;53(1):13-7.

Dalbayrak S, Onen MR, Yilmaz M, Naderi S. Clinical and radiographic results of balloon kyphoplasty for treatment of vertebral body metastases and multiple myelomas. J Clin Neurosci. 2010 Feb;17(2):219-24. Epub 2009 Dec 5.

Dashti H, Lee HC, Karaikovic EE, Gaines Jr RW. Decision making in thoracolumbar fractures. Neurol India 2005;53:534-41.

de Falco R, Scarano E, Di Celmo D, Grasso U, Guarnieri L. Balloon kyphoplasty in traumatic fractures of the thoracolumbar junction. Preliminary experience in 12 cases. J Neurosurg Sci. 2005 Dec;49(4):147-53.

Doria C, Tranquilli Leali P. Percutaneous techniques in the treatment of osteoporotic, traumatic and neoplastic fractures of thoraco-lumbar spine: our institutional experience. Injury. 2010 Nov;41(11):1136-9. Epub 2010 Oct 16

Furtado N, Oakland RJ, Wilcox RK, Hall RM. A biomechanical investigation of vertebroplasty in osteoporotic compression fractures and in prophylactic vertebral reinforcement. Spine (Phila Pa 1976). 2007 Aug 1;32(17):E480-7.

Gaitanis IN, Hadjipavlou AG, Katonis PG, Tzermiadianos MN, Pasku DS, Patwardhan AG. Balloon kyphoplasty for the treatment of pathological vertebral compressive fractures. Eur Spine J. 2005 Apr;14(3):250-60. Epub 2004 Oct 8.

Gaitanis IN, Hadjipavlou AG, Katonis PG, Tzermiadianos MN, Pasku DS, Patwardhan AG. Balloon kyphoplasty for the treatment of pathological vertebral compressive fractures. Eur Spine J. 2005 Apr;14(3):250-60. Epub 2004 Oct 8.

Gertzbein SD. Neurologic deterioration in patients with thoracic and lumbar fractures after admission to the hospital. Spine 1994;19:1723-5.

Greene DL, Isaac R, Neuwirth M, Bitan FD. The eggshell technique for prevention of cement leakage during kyphoplasty. J Spinal Disord Tech. 2007 May;20(3):229-32.

Groen RJ, du Toit DF, Phillips FM, Hoogland PV, Kuizenga K, Coppes MH, Muller CJ, Grobbelaar M, Mattyssen J. Anatomical and pathological considerations in percutaneous vertebroplasty and kyphoplasty: a reappraisal of the vertebral venous system. Spine (Phila Pa 1976). 2004 Jul 1;29(13):1465-71.

Grohs JG, Matzner M, Trieb K, Krepler P. Treatment of intravertebral pseudarthroses by balloon kyphoplasty. J Spinal Disord Tech. 2006 Dec;19(8):560-5.

Hide IG, Gangi A. Percutaneous vertebroplasty: history, technique and current perspectives. Clin Radiol 2004;59:461-7.

Hulme PA, Krebs J, Ferguson SJ, Berlemann U. Vertebroplasty and kyphoplasty: a systematic review of 69 clinical studies. Spine (Phila Pa 1976). 2006 Aug 1;31(17):1983-2001.

Jones JO, Bruel BM, Vattam SR. Management of painful vertebral hemangiomas with kyphoplasty: a report of two cases and a literature review. Pain Physician. 2009 Jul-Aug;12(4):E297-303.

Kalteis T, Lüring C, Gugler G, Zysk S, Caro W, Handel M, Grifka J. Acute tissue toxicity of PMMA bone cements. Z Orthop Ihre Grenzgeb. 2004 Nov-Dec;142(6):666-72.

Kalteis T, Lüring C, Gugler G, Zysk S, Caro W, Handel M, Grifka J. Acute tissue toxicity of PMMA bone cements. Z Orthop Ihre Grenzgeb. 2004 Nov-Dec;142(6):666-72.

Klazen CA, Lohle PN, de Vries J, Jansen FH, Tielbeek AV, Blonk MC, Venmans A, van Rooij WJ, Schoemaker MC, Juttmann JR, Lo TH, Verhaar HJ, van der Graaf Y, van Everdingen KJ, Muller AF, Elgersma OE, Halkema DR, Fransen H, Janssens X, Buskens E, Mali WP. Vertebroplasty versus conservative treatment in acute osteoporotic vertebral compression fractures (Vertos II): an open-label randomised trial. Lancet. 2010 Sep 25;376(9746):1085-92.

Kühn K-D. Bone Cements, Up-to-Date Comparison of Physicaland Chemical Properties of Commercial Materials. 2000 Springer Verlag: Berlin, pp. 12–20.

Lavelle W, Carl A, Lavelle ED, Khaleel MA. Vertebroplasty and kyphoplasty. Anesthesiol Clin. 2007 Dec;25(4):913-28.

Ledlie JT, Renfro MB. Kyphoplasty treatment of vertebral fractures: 2-year outcomes show sustained benefits. Spine (Phila Pa 1976). 2006 Jan 1;31(1):57-64.

Libicher M, Hillmeier J, Liegibel U, Sommer U, Pyerin W, Vetter M, Meinzer HP, Grafe I, Meeder P, Nöldge G, Nawroth P, Kasperk C. Osseous integration of calcium phosphate in osteoporotic vertebral fractures after kyphoplasty: initial results from a clinical and experimental pilot study. Osteoporos Int. 2006;17(8):1208-15. Epub 2006 Jun 8.

Luo J, Skrzypiec DM, Pollintine P, Adams MA, Annesley-Williams DJ, Dolan P. Mechanical efficacy of vertebroplasty: influence of cement type, BMD, fracture severity, and disc degeneration. Bone. 2007 Apr;40(4):1110-9. Epub 2007 Jan 16.

Magerl F, Aebi M, Gertzbein SD, Harms J, Nazarian S. A comprehensive classification of thoracic and lumbar injuries. Eur Spine J. 1994; 3(4):184-201.

Masala S, Fiori R, Massari F, Cantonetti M, Postorino M, Simonetti G. Percutaneous kyphoplasty: indications and technique in the treatment of vertebral fractures from myeloma. Tumori. 2004 Jan-Feb;90(1):22-6.

Mathis JM, Barr JD, Belkoff SM, et al. Percutaneous vertebroplasty: a developing standard of care for vertebral compression fractures. AJNR Am J Neuroradiol 2001;22(2):373-81

McKiernan F, Faciszewski T, Jensen R. Reporting height restoration in vertebral compression fractures. Spine (Phila Pa 1976). 2003 Nov 15;28(22):2517-21; discussion 3.

Molina GS, Campero A, Feito R, Pombo S. Kyphoplasty in the Treatment of Osteoporotic Vertebral Compression Fractures (VCF) : Procedure Description and Analysis of the Outcomes in 128 Patients. Acta Neurochir Suppl. 2011;108:163-170.

Movrin I, Vengust R, Komadina R. Adjacent vertebral fractures after percutaneous vertebral augmentation of osteoporotic vertebral compression fracture: a comparison of balloon kyphoplasty and vertebroplasty. Arch Orthop Trauma Surg. 2010 Sep;130(9):1157-66. Epub 2010 May 7.

Nairn RJ, Binkhamis S, Sheikh A. Current Perspectives on Percutaneous Vertebroplasty: Current Evidence/Controversies, Patient Selection and Assessment, and Technique and Complications. Radiology Research and Practice, vol. 2011, Article ID 175079, 10 pages, 2011. doi:10.1155/2011/175079

Oakland RJ, Furtado NR, Wilcox RK, Timothy J, Hall RM. Preliminary biomechanical evaluation of prophylactic vertebral reinforcement adjacent to vertebroplasty under cyclic loading. Spine J. 2009 Feb;9(2):174-81. Epub 2008 Jul 21.

Röllinghoff M, Zarghooni K, Schlüter-Brust K, Sobottke R, Schlegel U, Eysel P, Delank KS. Indications and contraindications for vertebroplasty and kyphoplasty. Arch Orthop Trauma Surg. 2010 Jun;130(6):765-74. Epub 2010 Mar 11.

Schmelzer-Schmied N, Cartens C, Meeder PJ, Dafonseca K. Comparison of kyphoplasty with use of a calcium phosphate cement and non-operative therapy in patients with traumatic non-osteoporotic vertebral fractures. Eur Spine J. 2009 May;18(5):624-9. Epub 2009 Jan 23.

Schwardt J, Slater T, Lee S, Meyer J, Wenz R. KyphOs FS™ Calcium Phosphate for Balloon Kyphoplasty: Verification of Compressive Strength and Instructions for Use. European Cells and Materials Vol. 11. Suppl. 1, 2006 (page 28).

Tseng YY, Yang TC, Tu PH, Lo YL, Yang ST. Repeated and multiple new vertebral compression fractures after percutaneous transpedicular vertebroplasty. Spine (Phila Pa 1976). 2009 Aug 15;34(18):1917-22.

Van Eenenaam DP, el-Khoury GY. Delayed post-traumatic vertebral collapse (Kummell's disease): case report with serial radiographs, computed tomographic scans, and bone scans. Spine (Phila Pa 1976). 1993 Jul;18(9):1236-41.

Verlaan JJ, van Helden WH, Oner FC, Verbout AJ, Dhert WJ. Balloon vertebroplasty with calcium phosphate cement augmentation for direct restoration of traumatic thoracolumbar vertebral fractures. Spine (Phila Pa 1976). 2002 Mar 1;27(5):543-8.

Wehrli FW, Ford JC, Haddad JG. Osteoporosis: clinical assessment with quantitative MR imaging in diagnosis. Radiology 1995;196(3):631–41.

Zoarski GH, Snow P, Olan WJ, Stallmeyer MJ, Dick BW, Hebel JR, De Deyne M. Percutaneous vertebroplasty for osteoporotic compression fractures: quantitative prospective evaluation of long-term outcomes. J Vasc Interv Radiol. 2002 Feb;13(2 Pt 1):139-48.

Zou J, Mei X, Gan M, Yang H. Kyphoplasty for spinal fractures from multiple myeloma. J Surg Oncol. 2010 Jul 1;102(1):43-7.

Anatomical and Surgical Perspective to Approach Degenerative Disc Hernias

H. Selim Karabekir[1], Nuket Gocmen-Mas[2] and Mete Edizer[3]
[1]Department of Neurosurgery, Kocatepe University School of Medicine, Afyonkarahisar,
[2]Department of Anatomy, Faculty of Medicine, Kocatepe University, Afyonkarahisar,
[3]Department of Anatomy, Faculty of Medicine, Dokuz Eylul University, Izmir,
Turkey

1. Introduction

The anatomy of the vertebral colomn is very important for neurosurgeons, orthopedists, traumatologists, neurologists, radiologists, anestesiologists and pathologists to aid in diagnosis, treatment, planning surgery, and the application of anesthesia or surgery (Winn, 2004).

Intervertebral discs are placed on between adjacent surfaces of vertebral bodies from axis to sacrum. There is no intervertebral disc between atlas and axis. The lowest functional intervertebral disc is located between fifth lumbar (L5) and sacrum. Thicknesses of the discs show variations in different regions and part of the same disc. They are thicker anteriorly and the anterior convexity is obvious in lumbar and cervical regions, but they are nearly uniform and the anterior concavity is large due to vertebral bodies in the thoracic region. In the upper thoracic region, discs are thinnest, but they thickest in the lumbar region. Intervertebral discs are avascular. They supplied by diffusion through the trabecular bone of nearby vertebrae. In brief, discs supplied from neighborhood blood vessels, except for their periphers. Vascular and avascular parts of discs show different reaction to injury.

Radicular damages related with degenerative disc hernias negatively affect innervation area of the spinal nerves, sensibility and ability of the patients to translate patterns of altered nerves activity into meaningful motor behaviors. The sensory or motor alterations can be attributed to functional or anatomical changes within the nerve roots after resolution of inflammation and edema and also surrounding of the nerves (Chaichana et al., 2011; Van Zundert et al., 2010; Lipetz, 2002).

2. Anatomy of vertebral column

2.1 Embriology

Vertebrae develop from the sclerotome parts of the somites, which are undergone, a change from the paraaxial mesoderm. A typical vertebra forms a vertebral arch and foramen, a body, transverse process, and usually a spinous process. Sclerotome cells move around the spinal cord and notochord to merge with cells from the opposing somite on the opposite side of the neural tube during the fourth week. As development continues, the sclerotome part of each somite also transposes a resegmentation. Resegmentation means as growing and blending of the caudal half of each sclerotome with the cephalic half of each subjacent sclerotome. So, each vertebra is combined between the caudal half of one somite and the cranial half of its neighbor. Modeling of the shapes of the different vertebrae is modulated by HOX genes (Sadler, 2006). Hox genes were defined to be involved in the manufacture of vertebrae with individual properties (Krumlauf 1994; Wellik 2007; Mallo et al., 2009). Mesenchymal cells which placed between two caudal parts of the sclerotome segment and fill the space between two precartilaginous vertebral bodies. In this way, they form the intervertebral discs. Although the notochord regresses entirely in the region of the vertebral bodies, it asserts and expands in the disc space. It supports the nucleus pulposus, which is covered loop shaped fibers of the annulus fibrosus. These two structures compose the intervertebral disc together (Sadler, 2006; Moore, 1992; Williams et al, 1995; Snell, 1997; April, 1990)

Resegmentation of sclerotomes into descriptive vertebrae cause the myotomes to bridge the intervertebral discs. This differentiation gains the discs spine motion capacity. Due to this development, intersegmental arteries, at first placed between the sclerotomes, to come to pass midway over the vertebral bodies (Sadler, 2006). Spinal nerves go to near the intervertebral discs and exit from the intervertebral foramina to leave vertebral column at that level (Moore, 1992; Williams et al, 1995; Snell, 1997; April, 1990).

2.2 Vertebral morphology

The vertebral column compose 33-34 number of vertebrae which are seven cervical, twelve thoracic, five lumbar vertebrae, a sacrum and three to five coccygeal vertebrae (Standrings et al, 2005; Williams et al, 1995). Each typical vertebra has a ventral body (except atlas) and dorsal vertebral arch, together enclosing a vertebral foramen. The adjacent bodies are attached together by intervertebral discs. The foramina form a vertebral canal for spinal cord. Intervertebral foramina which are located between adjoining vertebral arches, allow transmit spinal nerves, blood and lymphatic vessels. The vertebral body varies in size according to its level on vertebral column. The vertebral arch has one each side anteriorly the *pedicle*, and posteriorly the *lamina*. It also has paired transverse, superior and inferior articular processes and posteriorly a median spinous process. The pedicles are thick, short vertically narrower parts. Adjacent vertebral notches assist to an intervertebral foramen when vertebrae are articulated by the intervertebral discs. The laminae which directly continuous with pedicles are vertically broader flattened parts. The articular processes which are named as zygoapophyses joint compose paired superior and inferior articular processes. The superior ones locate on cranially, and the inferior ones caudally. Articular processes of adjoining vertebrae thus form synovial zygoapophyses joints together. These joints permit limited movement between vertebrae. The transverse processes project laterally. Only the thoracic transverse processes articulate with the ribs via their articular faces. The spinous process projects posteriorly and often caudally from the laminal junction. The spines vary in size, shape and directions according to vertebral level.

There are some regional features and differences of vertebrae. Vertebrae in different regions of the vertebral column show some modified characteristics from the typical pattern. There are conspicuous varieties in the size of the vertebral foramina in the same regions of different persons. There are also differences in the size and shape of the vertebral canal. These variations occur because of the spinal cord enlargements in the cervical and lumbosacral regions for the innervations of the limbs via plexuses (Moore, 1992).

Distinctive characterization of the cervical vertebrae is the oval shaped foramen transversarium. The vertebral arteries pass through the foramina in the transverse process, except those in prominent vertebra (C7) which lie only small accessory vertebral veins. Each of the processes has anterior and posterior tubercles on their upper surfaces. The groove for the spinal nerves locates between the tubercles from third cervical vertebra (C3) to C7 vertebrae, bilaterally. The anterior tubercle of sixth cervical vertebra (C6) which is named as carotic tubercle is bigger than the others. Due to large size of the tubercle, it may compress the common carotid artery. The spinous processes of C3 to C6 vertebrae are short and bifid. The spinous process of C7 is very long, so it is also important as an anatomical landmark for clinicians.

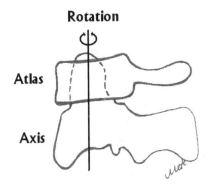

Fig. 1. The relationship between atlas and axis were shown while rotation (Illustrated by Edizer).

Atlas (C1) and axis (C2) are atypical vertebrae. C1 is a ring-shaped bone. The kidney-shaped, concave superior articular surfaces of C1 have the occipital condyles. The atlas has no spinous process or body; it has anterior and posterior arches. Each of the arch consists a tubercle and a lateral mass which is named as massa lateralis atlantis. C2 is named as axis and the skull rotates on it. The axis consists two large flat bearing the superior articular facets upon which the atlas rotates (Figure 1). Its distinguishing characteristic, however, is the blunt tooth-like dens which are called as odontoid process; place on superiorly from its body. The transverse ligament of the atlas supports dens for its position and prevents horizontal displacement of the atlas (Moore, 1992).

Distinctive features of the thoracic vertebrae are existance of the fovea costalis to articulate with the ribs (Figure 2). Adjoining upper and lower costal fovea and also intervertebral disc together articulate with fovea costalis of a rib. The thoracic vertebra has a small nearly oval foramen vertebra. The spinous processes of the thoracic vertebrae are long and slender. The middle ones are directed inferiorly over the vertebral arches of the inferior vertebrae to them. But the laminae are short, broad and thick. The spinous process is long and oblique shaped and lies inferiorly. The transverse processes which are large, strong and club-like, project from the vertebral arch at pediculolaminar junctions. They point dorsolaterally, near their apex, ventral oval facets articulating with tubercles of corresponding ribs. The eleventh and the twelfth thoracic vertebrae have not the costal tubercles.

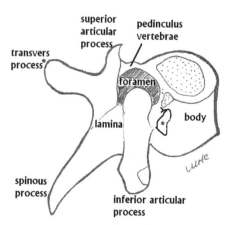

Fig. 2. Typical thoracic vertebra was shown (Illustrated by Edizer)

Differences of the lumbal vertebrae are their large size, absence of costal facets and transverse foramina (Moore, 1992). The body is big, thick and kidney shaped. The vertebral foramen is triangular shaped. The pedicles are short and the spinous process is nearly horizontal, quadrangular shaped and thick. L5 is distinct to its stout transverse processes. It is mostly amenable for the lumbosacral angle between the lumbar region and sacrum.

The sacrum which is fused by five vertebrae is a large, triangular shaped bone. It locates behind the pelvis and between two of the coxae. Its blunted, caudal tip articulates with the coccyx and its upper wide base articulates with the fifth lumbar vertebra. It consists dorsal, pelvic and lateral surfaces and a sacral canal between the apex and the base. Anterior projecting edge of the base is the sacral promontory. Four pairs of anterior sacral foramina place on the pelvic (anterior) surface. The ventral rami of the upper four sacral spinal nerves transmit through intervertebral foramina with the sacral canal via the pelvic sacral foramina. Similarly, four pairs of dorsal sacral foramina locate on the dorsal surface. The lateral surface projects as a broad articular part. Its upper parts have auricular surfaces, bilaterally. The sacral canal forms by sacral vertebral foramina. Its caudal opening is called as sacral hiatus. The canal contains the cauda equina including its flum terminale and spinal meninges. The coccyx is a small triangle bone. It usually consists of three to five fused rudimentary vertebrae (Williams et al, 1995; Moore, 1992).

As a conclusion the vertebral architecture is significant as it combine stability, load-bearing capacity and motor function and also covers contained neurovascular structures such as vessels, spinal nerves, irrespective of its position (Williams et al, 1995). Regional variants can see in mobility of the verterbrae on the geometry, position, placement and properties of both zygoapophysial joints and related ligaments around the column. The ligament flava, interspinous, supraspinous and posterior longitudinal ligaments and posterior margin of intervertebral disc are tensed, interlaminar intervals wider, inferior facet glide on superior facet of subjacent vertebrae and their capsules become taut.

2.3 Intervertebral disc morphology

The discs are composed of circular anuli fibrosi covering gelatinous nuclei pulposi. The anuli fibrosi insert into compact bony edges on articular face of the vertebral bodies. It has a narrow outer collagen zone and a wider inner fibrocartiloginous zone. The annulus fibrosus consists of concentric lamellae of collagenous fibers which lie obliquely from one vertebra to the other (Figure 3). The lamellae are less numerous posteriorly and thinner than they are anteriorly and laterally. The nuclei pulposi contact the hyaline articular cartilages, which are attached to endplates of the bodies. It is large, soft and gelatinous and mucoid materials with a multinucleated notochordal cell at birth. The cells disappeare in the first decade followed by gradual replacement of mucoid material by fibrocartilage derivated principally from the annulus fibrosus and the hyaline cartilaginous plates adjoining vertebral bodies. The nucleus pulposus is better developed in cervical and lumbar regions. It behaves toward like shock absorber for axial forces and like water bed bearing during flexion, extension and lateral bending of the vertebral column. The water content of nucleus pulposus is about 88% and its turgor and also fullness is great in the young adults. Discs are more often damaged by twisting and flexing the vertebral column. The intervertebral discs are so strong that violence first damages the neighborhood bone in young adults. It is possible to damage a healthy disc by forcible flexion as well as extension. Degenerative changes on discs may result in necrosis, sequestration of the nucleus pulposus, weakening or softening of annulus fibrosus after second decade. Then minor strains may cause internal disharmony with eccentric displacement of the nucleus pulposus. The minor strains may also cause external disharmony. In this case, the nucleus pulposus than bulges through annulus fibrosus may occur usually posterolaterally. The discs are also show pathological changes that may result in protrusion of nucleus pulposus through the annulus fibrosus known as a herniated or prolapsed disc. As people getting older, the nuclei pulposi lose their turgor and become thinner due to degeneration and dehydration. Symptom producing disc herniations happen in the cervical region almost as in the lumbar region. In geriatric ages, degenerative changes may occur in the discs because of relatively minor stress.

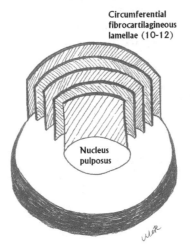

Fig. 3. Structural demonstration of an intervertebral disc (Illustrated by Edizer).

The discs support by anterior and posterior longitudinal ligaments. These ligaments lie throughout vertebral column. The anterior longitudinal ligament holds on the vertebral bodies strongly, but it adheres to the intervertebral disc tenderly. It originates from occipital bone and lies to sacral canal. Despite to anterior longitudinal ligament, the posterior longitudinal ligament which is the principal, but narrow ligament of intervertebral discs to each other adheres to the intervertebral discs strongly. The posterior surface of the vertebral bodies have a little concave shape, so while the posterior longitudinal ligament lies from one body to the other adhere with loose connective tissue in the canal (Figure 4) (Moore, 1992; Williams et al,1995 ; Snell, 1997; April, 1990).

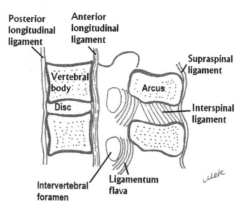

Fig. 4. Vertebral column and related ligaments were shown (Illustrated by Edizer).

2.4 Spinal nerve morphology

There are 31 pairs of the spinal nerves as eight cervical, twelve thoracic, five lumbar, five sacral and a coccygeal, bilaterally. They originate through intervertebral foramina for each level. However, the first spinal nerve leaves the vertebral canal between atlas and the occipital bone, bilaterally. So, the nerve is named as the suboccipital nerve. Each of the nerve is continous with the spinal cord by the anterior (ventral) and posterior (dorsal) roots, the latter each bearing a spinal ganglion (Taner D, 2004; Van de Graaf, 1998; Williams et al, 1995; Moore, 1992). The anterior roots compose axons of neurons in the anterior and lateral spinal grey columns. The posterior roots also contain centripedal process of neurons sited in the spinal ganglia. The spinal nerves have clinically significant relations in the vertebral foramina. The relations are anteriorly, with the intervertebral discs and adjacent vertebral bodies. Posterior are the zygapophysial joints. Superior and inferior are vertebral notches of the pedicles of adjoining vertebrae. Each of the spinal nerve accompanied by a spinal artery, a small venous plexus and its meningeal branch or branches together traverse a foramen (Williams et al, 1995). Dorsal (posterior) rami of spinal nerves, usually smaller than the ventral (anterior) and directed posteriorly divide into medial and lateral branches (except for the first cervical, fourth and fifth sacral and coccygeal nerves) to innervate the muscles and skin of the posterior regions of the neck and trunk. The ventral rami of spinal nerves innervate the limbs and the anterolateral aspect of the trunk, they are mostly larger than the dorsal rami. The thoracic nerves are independent and retain, like all dorsal rami, mostly segmental distirubition. The cervical, lumbar and sacral spinal nerves connect near their origins to form plexuses like cervical plexus in cervical region, brachial plexus in lower cervical and thoracic region and lumbosacral plexus in lumbosacral region, which are called as the peripheric nerves. Dorsal rami do not join these plexuses (Williams et al, 1995).

The spinal nerves might be compressed by herniated discs. Because of the protrusion and compression, the patients suffer from chronic pain symptom. All symptoms and signs occure usually on the same side as the herniation but sometimes the cases have contralateral side pain symptom, which leads to the fact that operators are in doubt about the decision to perform disc surgery. In the literature the possible mechanism of contralateral pain symptoms may occure due to hyperthrophy of ligamenta flava (Karabekir et al 2010). So, surgeons should take care for anatomical landmarks releated with ligamentous complex during surgery.

3. Degenerative disc hernias

3.1 Description and scope

Degenerative disc disease (DDD) occurs when the outer ring, annulus fibrosus, damaged of worn. The contents of the disc may then protrude or impinge on a spinal root. This will cause pain in the lower back and that radiates to the hips and down the back of the legs. Backpain is an unpleasent and noxius sensation of varying severity localized in different regions of the back. The simplified etiologic or pathogenetic classification of back pain includes myofascial, articular (including degenerative disc changes), and neurogenic components. Because of increased incidance of low back pain (LBP) or lumbosacral radicular syndrome, low back pain becomes a serious problem for healthy and active individuals between the ages 30-50.

If a degenerative disc hernia is obtained then simple discectomy is offered to the individuals. Neverthless there are some problems followed by degenerative disc disease operations such as recurrence, loss of height and instability. The most effective treatment of discogenic pain to unresponsive to conservative care is interbody fusion in the literature (Karabekir et al, 2008).

The development of molecular biology enabled a better understanding of the processes that caused the degenerative disease of intervertebral discs. Many studies aiming to clarify the causes and risk factors for this degenerative disorder have been performed (Patel et al, 2007). It is now known that degenerative disc disease is strongly correlated to genetic factors, investigations indicating that heredity has a major role for degeneration of disc and implies approximately 74% in adult populations, as a variation. Since 1998 there were many genes associated with degenerative disc hernias declarated such as MMP-3, VDR, collagen I, collagen IX (COL9A2 and COL9A3), collagen XI (COL11A2), vitamin D receptor, IL-1, IL-6, CILP, and aggrecan (Cevei et al 2011).

When the outer ring, annulus fibrosus, damage because of aging and/or degeneration, the degenerative disc disease occure (Figure 5). Then, the contents of the disc may protrude or impinge on a spinal root, unilaterally or sometimes bilaterally. This process will cause pain in the lower back and that radiates to the hips and down the back of the legs. At the same time degenerative disc disease may cause to segmental instability due to following ligamentous laxity, fall in the amount of the nucleus pulposus, and loss of disc height.

Segmental instability which appears as aberrant vertebral motion may be accountable for the pain. Low back pain may arise from the facet joints, but various clinical outcomes have not verified this theory (Marks et al, 1992; Schwarzerger et al, 1994; 1994).

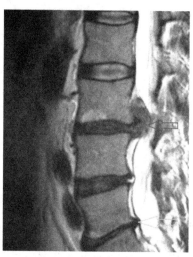

Fig. 5. An extrude disc hernia was shown by the red arrow and degenerative disc hernia was shown by the yellow one

Low back pain can unpleasantly appear in different regions of the back. The pathogenetic classification of low back pain divides into three types as myofascial, articular (including degenerative disc changes), and neurogenic. Back pain can cause several problems. It can effect healthy, active individuals between 30 and 50 years old. Invasive treatment options for chronic LBP are mostly tried after conservative cures have failed to obtain the desired results (Buric et al, 2011). Fusion and total disc arthroplasty are the most frequent surgical procedure to treat LBP caused by DDD with or without segmental instability. Nonetheless, the clinical achievement of fusion varies widely (16–95%) and to relate principally with the indication value being used (Turner et al, 1992; 1993; Waddel et al, 2000). Cases who undergo spinal fusions or total disc replacement mostly have more complications, longer stay in hospital and higher charges from hospital than cases undergoing other types of operation. LBP is usually resulting from mechanical reasons like load, which may initiate internal disc degeneration and trigger loss of water from the nucleus pulposus. The consecutive step of degenerative episode gives rise to a decline in disc height, narrowing of the intervertebral space, and non-organized facet joints. These episodes disturb anatomical and physiological motion between two neighborhood vertebrae and increase instability due to laxity of the ligaments and the annulus fibrosus (Buric et al, 2011).

Modic firstly delineated classifications of lumbar spine degeneration via imaging technique (Hutton et al, 2011). The author classified the cases as grade I, II or III using MRI. According to his follow up results, MRI changes compose of vertebral bodies parallel with the vertebral plateau of degenerated disc which indicates hyposignal on the slices in T1 and hyperintensity in T2 for Type I. The changes of MRI composed of rised intensity of the signal on the images in T1 and an isointense signal or lightly hyperintense in T2 and represent the imagistic expression of disc lesions consisting of annular protrusion and comparatively recent initial beginning disc hernia for Type II. Both Type I and II have not a radiological correspondent. MRI investigations revealing type III changes, represent decreasing intensity of the signal on the slices both in T1 and T2, being related on regular planar radiographic slices with extensive bone sclerosis. Those changes are related with disc extrusion, disc hernia, free disc fragment, problems of the posterior vertebral ligament (Gocmen-Mas, 2010; Karabekir et al, 2010). The composition of the disc changes during development, growth, ageing and degeneration and this impress the response of the disc to changes in mechanical stress (Cevei et al 2011; Modic, 2007).

Diagnosis of degenerative disc disease is confirmed by MRI scans (West et al, 2010). Direct x-rays, especially planar flexion-extension radiographies may help to recognize instability which develops because of degenerative disc disease. Discography is also important for diagnostic survey of the degenerative disc disease.

4. Treatment modalities of degenerative disc hernias

4.1 Surgical procedures

In biomechanical respect posterior lumbar interbody fusion (PLIF), introduced by Dr.Ralph Cloward in the 1940.s, is an optimal fusion. A succesful PLIF carries the advantages of immobilizing the unstable degenerated intervertebral disc area, decompressing the dural sac and nerve roots, restoring disc height and load bearing to anterior structures. In spite of a lot of fusion techniques, such as autologous iliac crest bone graft, allograft bone, dowelshaped graft, key stone graft, tricortical graft, and bone chips, interbody cages preferred. There is various types of cages, carbon-titanium-polyetherether keton etc., are used for interbody fusion (Figure 2-5). In our daily practice we prefered polyetherether keton (PEEK) cages because of their safety usage and wide graft space contains (Karabekir et al, 2009).

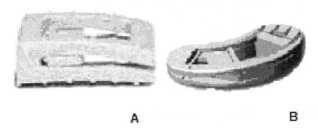

A   B

Fig. 6. Samples of expandable PEEK cages; A. Cervical, B. Lumbal

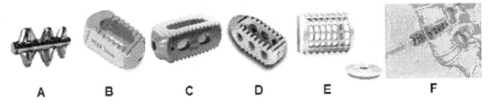

A   B   C   D   E   F

Fig. 7. Samples of the intervertebral cages; A. B-twin, B. B-D PEEK cages, E-F. Cylendiric titanium cages.

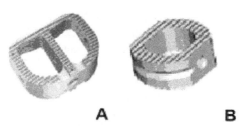

A   **B**

Fig. 8. Samples of the cervical PEEK cages (A and B)

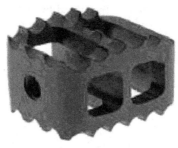

Fig. 9. A sample of the carbon intervertebral cage

PLIF usually has been accomplished with implantation of two threaded cages (Bagby, 1988). The rate of fusion of bone grafts alone have ranged from 46% to 90% at the literature. Because of difficulty in maintaining spinal stabilization and achieving fusion, spinal instrumentation has become an important and popular adjunct to bone grafting in lumbar arthrodesis, further increasing the fusion rates, 80-90% (Karabekir et al, 2009).

More recently, interbody fusion techniques have also shown high fusion rates with distinct advantages (Lin et al, 1983; Ray, 1997). Some of these advantages include immediate anterior column load sharing, a large surface area for fusion, bone graft subjected to compressive loads that is advantegous in achieving fusion and the ability to restore normal sagittal contour while indirectly decompressing the intervertebral foramen (Lin et al, 1983). Interbody fusion technique also appear to be the most effective cure of discogenic back pain unresponsive to conservative care (Weatherly et al, 1986).

Blume, in 1981, described a unilateral approach for posterior lumbar interbody fusion to address some of the potential complications of the standart PLIF such as spinal nerves' roots injuries, and instabilization. The unilateral posterior lumbar interbody fusion (UPLIF) popularized by Harms et al (1997) is a surgical technique in which bilateral anterior column support can be achieved through a unilateral posterior approach.

Weatherly et al (1986) reported on five cases during a 10-year period who had solid posterolateral fusions, but still had positive discography under the fusion and had their back pain relieved by anterior interbody fusion.

Recently, Derby et al (1999) noted that cases with highly sensitive discs as determined by pressure controlled discography achieved significantly better long-term outcomes with combined anterior and posterior fusion.

Nevertheless, there are some problems followed by degenerative disc disease operations such as recurrence, lost of height and instability. Many authors develop some different surgical approaches for preventing the recurrence of disc herniation and to protect the disc height. Of these modified techniques, we prefer, in our daily practice consists of unilateral and bilateral polyetheretherketon (PEEK) posterior lumbar cages by using demineralized bone matrix (DBM) putty graft (Karabekir et al, 2008).

UPLIF is indicated for chronic mechanical pain associated with degenerative disc disease, recurrent disc herniation. With this concept recurrence of disc and the possibility of foraminal narrowing and loss of height can also be reduced. The most advantage of the PEEK cage is to preserve the disc space height and prevent the recurrence. Unilateral posterior PEEK cage application and fusion is a safe and reproducible technique to provide unilateral posterior column support (Karabekir et al, 2009). With this method, recurrence of the disc and the possibility of foraminal narrowing and loss of height can also be reduced (Karabekir et al 2008).

Although PLIF has shown satisfactory clinical outcomes in treatment of degenerative disc diseases, many studies have reported that accelerated adjacent segment degeneration (ASD) may occur after PLIF management, particularly at the rostral level (Kumar et al., 2001; Okuda et al., 2008; Park et al., 2004; Zencica et al., 2010; Chen et al., 2011).

There is controversial relationship between fusion surgery and adjacent segment degeneration. Battie et al (2004) declared that adjacent segment degeneration after fusion was a natural status that was not associated to the fusion surgery. However, some other investigators implied in vitro mechanical studies and found that lumbar fusion may increase abnormal intradiscal pressure and too much movement at the adjacent spinal levels, resulting in adjacent segment degeneration (Lee et al, 2009). Therefore, it appears that adjacent segment disease may be especially caused by the abnormal discal stresses distribution that occurred by lumbar fusion and fixation. The other serious complication of posterior fixation and fusion operations is damaging of the nerve roots because of the placement of pedicular implants from the posterior (Ebrahaim et al, 1997). And also neuropathic pain associated with implant placement is not rare in literature. In the implantology literature, complications related to nerve are mentioned as 'sensory disturbances', focusing on the occurrence of paresthesia and dysesthesia, eventually accompanied by transitory pain sensations during implant placement (Ebrahaim et al, 1997; Butt et al, 2007).

DDD and its related symptoms have classically been cured with spinal fusion where the affected vertebrae are immobilized with mechanical fasteners or cages. This method stabilizes the impressed segments and achieved pain recipe (Balsano et al, 2011; Gornet et al, 2011).

A modified PLIF method named as transforaminal lumbar interbody fusion (TLIF), was first definated in 1982. Because the bone graft can be inserted far laterally, the TLIF technique can be safely indicated for interbody fusion of the upper lumbar spine. Moreover, TLIF can be performed at any lumbar level below first lumbar vertebra (L1), because it avoids significant retraction of the dura and conus medullaris (Hioki et al, 2011).

The minimally invasive lateral transpsoas method to the lumbar spine such as extreme lateral interbody fusion (XLIF) and direct lateral interbody fusion (DLIF) occurs as an alternative to interbody placement at levels L1 to L5 in the setting of spondylolisthesis, degenerative disc disease, and scoliotic or kyphotic anomalies (Benglis et al, 2008; Bergey et al, 2004; Cox et al, 2008; Dezawa et al, 2000; Mayer, 1997; Mc Afee et al 1998; Benglis et al, 2009).

But all of these approaches are not without complications. Outcomes of spinal fusion in a decreased range of movement and might caused a degenerative series in adjacent vertebral segments (Rahms, 1996). There have been many efforts to substitute the disc via various equipments for avoiding this and treating cases leaving its usual anatomic and physiologic movement (Balsano et al, 2011).

Recently, spinal movement preservation has so important in spine surgery as a potential planning to arrange a more normal spinal motion and providing against the biomechanical stress and a kinematic strain on nearby segments (Junjie et al, 2011). For protecting spinal motion an alternative to spinal fusion, total disc replacement (TDR) intervention is more and more becoming an adopted alternative for cases with degenerative disc disease. Theorically, the surgery carries on various benefits over spinal fusion, as it is desired to preserve mobilization and may diminish adjacent level degeneration. But, failures can make revision surgery a necessity for all kind of implant surgeries. McAfee et al (2009) report 8.8% revision procedures at the index level. Retrification of artificial discs is candidate to complications, because of revision surgery carries individual major risks for cases. McAfee et al (2009) claimed that a 3.6% incidence of vascular injury in primary TDR and 16.7% in anterior revision surgery. Revision surgery is usually applied to the cases with persistent severe low back pain or leg pain. This pain may releate with implant as malpositioning, prosthesis migration, subluxation, subsidence, and breakage of the metal ring of the core or wear.

Owing to adhesions, vascular structures are more vulnerable and adherent to the spine. Major vascular structures are placed on front to the discs at levels above L5 to S1. The vena cava and the aortic bifurcation mainly lie superior to the L5 to S1 disc levels, so the vascular complications give rise to anxiety. Other potential various complications are ureteral damage of the neural prevertebral plexus.

However, no definite proof of its biomechanical and clinical efficacy has yet been provided stand-alone devices are threaded cages designed for anterior lumbar interbody fusion (ALIF). Therefore all the instrument sets are designed for a wide approach to the disc. Moreover, additional space is required for to keep a regular distance between the vertebral endplates throughout the entire procedure by the working tube. The outer diameter of the smallest cage is 12 milimeters; the additional 2–3 mm of the working tube diameter would require about 15 mm of minimal working space on either side (Costa et al, 2011). Using these stand-alone cages is limited because they can be used only for discs which do not exceed 10 mm in height. Furthermore, these cages are suitable for any interbody fusion associated with pedicle screw fixation.

Nuclear replacement began with implantation of devices into the intervertebral disc space following discectomy. Pioneer prostheses contain stainless steel balls, self-curing silicone, silicone-Dacron composite, and polymethylmethacrylate. Other unsuccessful mechanical implants including springs and pistons have been developed. Most of these implants have been unsuccessful because of some complications such as extrusion, subsidence, and reactive endplate changes. Edeland (1981) implied that a nuclear implant should have viscoelastic features and permit influx and egress of water, thereby mimicking normal disc behaviors. The prosthetetic disc nucleus (PDN) prosthesis consist a capsule of woven polyethylene enclosing a hydroscopic thixotropic gel. Various similar products, which have including sheaths with elastic elements, have been tested but none are accepted. Another concept has been to directly inject hydrogel polymers such as polyvinyl alcohol into the intervertebral disc space. Water absorption and subsequent material expansion prevent protrusion. Nuclear replacement theorically restores degenerative disc biomechanics by changing height and at the same time effect the anular tension.

Symptomatic cases with soft disc hernia or moderate degenerative disc disease may be reckoned for TDR. Few investigations on the intervention of TDR in cervical spondylosis have been declared in literature (Byran VE, 2002; Lafuente et al, 2005; Pimenta et al, 2007; Sekhon LHS 2004), but concern remains on reasonable, efficacy, suitable and safety of disc prostheses in cases with multilevel spondylotic status of the cervical spine, due to accompanied facet joints differency and segmental bony degenerative alterations. The anterior cervical discectomy and fusion (ACDF) is the most largely accepted intervention for the cases with single or double level spondylotic disease. It has acceptable clinical outcomes and radiological fusion ranging from 90 to 100% are frequently cured either by anterior decompression and fusion (Matz et al, 2007), with (Mummaneni et al, 2007; Kaiser et al, 2002) cases with multilevel, symptomatic, spondylotic myeloradiculopathy or without plating (Ashkenazi et al, 2005) or by posterior decompression with or without lateral mass screw fixation (Wiggins et al, 2007). ACDF, a suitable and reliable method, is accepted as the gold standard intervention for single or multilevel cervical spondylosis to cause radiculopathy or myelopathy. It is not absolute whether or not anterior cervical discectomy is due to the physiological senescence of the spine or changes on the ground that previous fusion (Hilibrand et al, 2004). Fusion may be related with other causes such as pseudoarthrosis (Albert et al, 2004), donor site complications and factors of the neighborhood motion segments' biomechanics. The hybrid, single stage, fusion–nonfusion technique appears to be a promising and viable alternation in the treatment of symptomatic multilevel cervical DDD with prevalent anterior myeloradicular compression and different severity per single level, particularly in younger patients. It allows protecting or healing motion in some segments without defining iatrogenic spine instability or painful secondary to severely degenerated levels. Long-term follow-up on larger series of cases are need to approve all of the results (Barbagallo et al, 2009).

Presently there are two types of disc prosthesis as total disc and nucleus disc equipments (Bao et al, 2002; Bao et al, 2007; Bertagloni et al, 2003, Hedman et al 1991). Contrary to total disc replacement, nucleus disc prosthesis protects the existing constitutions, where include the ligaments, annulus, and endplates (Enker et al, 1993; Fernstrom 1966; Kostuik 1997). Nowadays, there are several types and designs of nucleus disc equipments, and surgical applications such as Nubactm which is the first articulating nucleus disc. Given that the mainly avascular intervertebral disc bears some of the highest loads in the human body and it is not surprising that DDD is a common phenomenon in middle age and a universal condition of the inevitable consequences of aging (Rothman et al 1982). The broad majority of cases achieve acceptable clinical outcomes without surgery (Weinstein, 1992). However, some cases do not respond to nonsurgical treatments. Chronically malformated cases population surgery may be useful. DDD and its related signs have classically been cured with spinal fusion. This method results in a diminished range of movement and may caused a degenerative process in adjacent vertebral segments (Lee CK, 1998; Ray, 1997; Lee CK et al, 1991; Nachemson, 1992; Kuslisch et al 1998). For a long time, fusion was reckoned as the gold standard of surgical procedure. However, clinical outcomes have yielded the acceptance of disc arthroplasty as the cure option (Balsano et al, 2011).

Several types of prosthesis have been planned with frequent improvements. The polyethylene core of the Charite´ prosthesis is sensitive to wear and hurts with breakage of the metal wire marker whether or not associated with impingement. This polyethylene wear gives rise to third-body debris in the intervertebral space near the spinal canal, which may lead to vertebral osteolysis. Retrieval surgery of Charite´ TDRs is convenient and relatively reliable, it has major risks due to adjacent vessels and scar tissue. Removal of keeled TDRs like Prodisc and Maverick implants is more hard and more bone removal is a necessity when above L5-S1 levels so, a lateral approach is preffered to avoid damage the major vascular structures (Gerardus et al, 2009). In our series we generally used porus coated motion (PCM) type cervical prosthesis and recently M-6 cervical disc prosthesis at cervical levels, and Nubac at lumbar regions.

The significant cause of recurrent low back pain after TDR may be facet degeneration or adjacent degeneration. The features of intervertebral disc prosthesis with articulating properties like long endurance are so important (Gerardus et al, 2009). The artificial disc or prosthesis is composed of critical importance to prevent premature disintegration; the artificial disc should generate a normal or near-normal movement compared with the pattern of healthy human spinal motion segment, so that corresponding facet joints and adjacent level or levels are not overloaded; and long-term fixation is necessary to avoid subsidence or migration. It seems almost impossible to provide a disc prosthesis that possesses all these features.

Disc arthroplasty provides a new concept not only in the cure of DDD but also in researching its biomechanics on anatomical changes and pathologies of the spine. Disc arthroplasty may fill the gap between simple discectomy and fusion concepts (Fekete et al, 2010).

A less invasive procedure, which is nowadays proposed for the management of chronic lumbar pain due to degenerative discopathy, involves the implantation of dynamic interspinous fixation devices (Bono et al 2007).

Lumbar interspinous spacers (ISPs) have recently become popular as an alternative treatment for lumbar DDD. Several spacers X-STOP, Coflex, Wallis, and DIAM are currently available and there have been various proposed indications (Figure 6). In the literature largest number of studies has been with the X-STOP device. The biomechanical studies with all the devices showed that ISPs have a beneficial effect on the kinematics of the degenerative spine. Apart from two randomized controlled trials, the other studies with the X-STOP device were not of high methodological quality (Kabir et al, 2011). Nevertheless, analysis of those studies showed that X-STOP may improve outcome when compared to non-operative cure in selected cases whose aged 50 or over, with radiologically confirmed lumbar canal stenosis and neurogenic claudication, who have improvement of their symptoms in flexion. Studies on the other interspinous devices show satisfactory outcome to varying degrees. However, due to small number and poor design of the studies, it is difficult to clearly define indications for ISP's use in lumbar degenerative disease. Lumbar ISPs may have a potential beneficial effect in selective cases with degenerative disease of the lumbar spine. However, further evidence based and good quality trials are needed to clearly outline the indications for ISP's use.

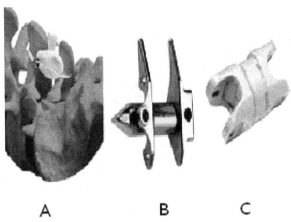

A   B   C

Fig. 10. Samples of the interspinous devices; A.Diam, B.X-Stop, C.PEEK interspinous devices

Nowadays advances in minimally invasive spine surgery (MISS) have allowed spinal surgeons to treat a broader range of degenerative spinal disorders. This is due to the development of advanced technology and new ways of approaching the spine. Some of the many factors that have driven these developments are the request of patients and spinal surgeons to lessen the morbidity and improve the outcome associated. Percutaneous axial anterior lumbar spine surgery is a possible and safe technique (Aryan et al, 2008). This technique is made feasible by a union of established spine surgery principles and the new technology of minimally invasive spinal surgery. The technique is important because it permits the implantation of biomechanically sound implants without the morbidity encountered in open surgery or other types of minimally invasive posterolateral spinal surgery (Aryan et al, 2007). The access orientation makes disc surgery with minimally invasive instruments more intuitive and accomplish. This technique will permit a routine percutaneous fusion from a single access site without paraspinal dissection and will lend itself to the development of new minimally invasive implant. This annulus fibrosus preserving and muscle-sparing approach will moderate postoperative pain, avoid postoperative scarring, speed healing, and eliminate problems encountered with annulus removal. This technique lends itself to spicing biomechanical solutions for motion preservation. Also, therapeutic interbody implants that can be replaced, expanded and revised easily will satisfy the patient and spine surgeon with a novel range of treatment options. The percutaneous paracoccygeal approach to the L5-S1 and L4-L5 interspaces provide a minimally invasive corridor through which discectomy and interbody fusion can safely be actualized. This approach can be used alone or in combination with minimally invasive or classical open fusion procedures. The technique may provide a disjunctive route of access to the L5-S1 or L4-L5 interspaces or both in those patients who may have aberrant anatomy for or contraindications to classical open anterior approach to this level (Aryan et al, 2008). Still this study does not provide Class 1 data, and is subject to the bias of any retrospective series, and further investigation beyond retrospective analysis is warranted before recommending the routine use of this technique.

Another technique can use after simple discectomy for preventing disc height. It also provides to replace a new injectable synthetic nucleus pulposus material instead of degenerative nucleus pulposus. Nucleus pulposus replacement is a non-fusion technique currently being investigated to treat painful disc degeneration. Replacement of nucleus pulposus with an injectable implant or tissue engineered construct, in patients with healthy annulus fibrosus, may reduce pain while simultaneously restoring spinal mobility and delaying disc degeneration (Boyd et al, 2006; Di Martino et al, 2005; Joshi et al, 2005; Klara et al, 2002; Larson et al, 2006; Cloyd et al, 2007). The challenge for any synthetic nucleus replacement material is to mimic the function of native nucleus pulposus. This bio-adhesive hydrogel material is one of the samples of these kinds of surgical materials (Cloyd et al, 2007; Gloria et al, 2010). After using these materials there's adhesions around the application site could observed. And a question related with application of these materials is the amount of these materials. This can be measured as weight at the operating room after discectomy by measuring the weight of the excising disc material.

Surgeons can measure the cages dimension preoperatively, but there's an easy and unbiased method that can be used before surgery. With this simple volume analysis technique surgeons can calculate how many cc disc material take place at intervertebral space and after discectomy the surgeons can calculate how many cc graft or bioglue substance can be necessary to put this space and what will be the dimensions of the cage or cages to put intervertebral disc space (Karabekir et al, 2011).

The stereological volume analysis is simple, reliable, unbiased and inexpensive. Intervertebral space volumes can evaluate using stereological method. A uniform point-grid with a point-associated area of 0.156 cm^2 is randomly superimposed on each MRI using the "Grid". Points hitting the lumbar intervertebral space are manually counted for area estimation of the profiles. Automated area estimation by manual perimeter tracing is generally take too much time and hence, more rapid point counting method is preferred. Volume estimation is accomplished by the Cavalieri's principle as described previously using the formula given below:

$$V = t \times [((SU \times d)/ SL]^2 \times {}_\Sigma P$$

where t is the section thickness, SU is the scale unit, d is the distance between two points in the point grid, SL is the scale length and $\sum P$ is the number of points counted. SU and SL are used to include the linear magnification in the final estimate. All data have been entered to a previously prepared Microsoft Excel spread sheet for automatic calculation of both the results of the above formula and the statistical evaluation parameters including the nugget variance and the coefficient of error (CE). All measurements are performed blinded to subject details and the results of any other measurements, and are done three times in each trial for inter-observer analysis by different researchers.

The surgeons can calculate the intervertebral space volume and discectomy material amount before surgery using this unbiased and inexpensive method (Karabekir et al, 2011). So while operating the cases the surgeons can use the correct amounts of materials and the materials which have correct dimensions.

4.2 Illustrative cases

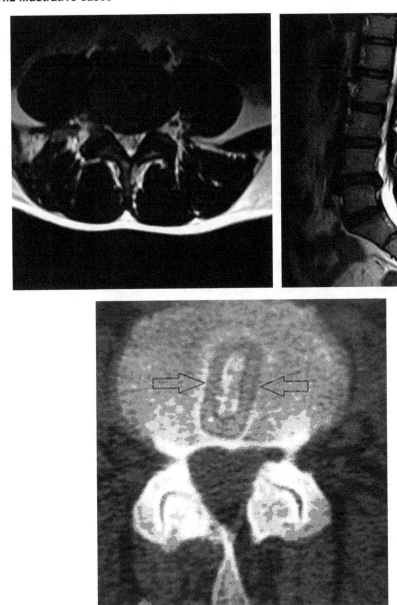

Fig. 11. Preoperative MRI and postoperative CT of 52-year old female case with degenerative disc disease were shown: The patient was admitted with left radicular leg pain and numbness. At physical examination loss of left L5 sensation and left dorsoflexion deficit were obtained. She was operated from left side and after discectomy unilateral PEEK cage was placed on L4-L5 levels (Karabekir, 2006). She had no complaint at 5 years follow-up.

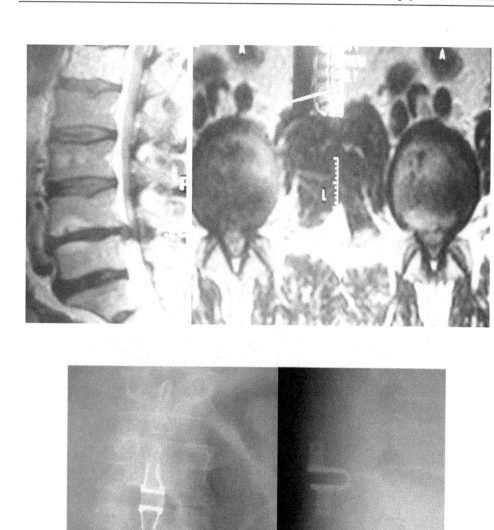

Fig. 12. L4-L5 diffuse protrusion and bilateral foraminal stenosis on preoperative MRI of a 55 year old men, whom had low back and bilateral leg pain which dominate at right side with numbness and causalgia during last 6 months, was shown. At physical examination bilateral muscle weakness at ankle dosoflexion and L4-S1 hypoesthesia were obtained. Postoperative anteroposterior and lateral X-rays of the case was shown. The interspinous device (Coflex) was applied at L4-L5 level after discectomy posteriorly to preserve the height of the interspinal foramens (Karabekir, 2005).

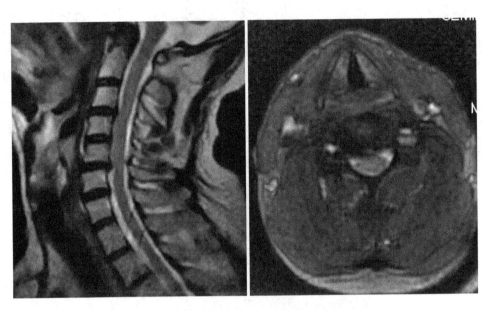

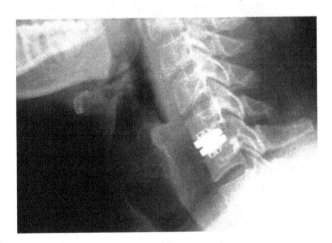

Fig. 13. Preoperative servical MRI was shown with C5-C6 servical degenerative disc hernia. 39 year-old male subject was admitted with right arm pain and numbness for three months period. At physical examination left C5-6-7 sensation lost, muscle weakness and biceps reflex hipoactivity were observed. Patient was operated and applicated Maverick artificial disc prosthesis at C5-C6 level (Karabekir, 2010). Artficial disk was shown at postoperative direct x-ray.

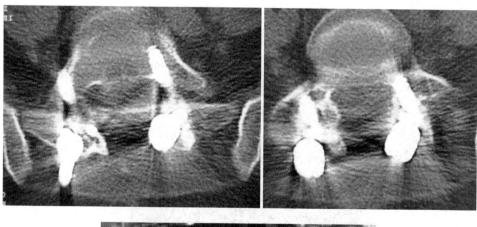

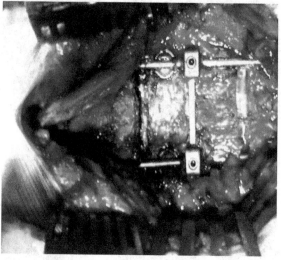

Fig. 14. Peroperative image of 64-year old female revision case; 3rd operation of the case, first simple discectomy and interbody fusion, the second posterior pedicle screws implantation because of chronic lowback pain and the third was performed because of broken screws. Broken screws were shown at W-B pictures (Karabekir, 2008).

5. Expert suggestions

The cases of degenerative disc disease should be evaluated carefully preoperatively and at operative period. The surgeon should know topographic and clinic anatomical knowledge of the region in detailed. Critical important anatomical landmarks should be defined before surgical approach such as lateral border of ligamentum flava and posterior longitudinal ligament, medial margin of superior articular process (superior facet). At the time of preoperative planning and during surgery; surgeon should aim to perform limited invasive procedure for preserving neighbourhood tissue and neurovascular structures of the region. Meticulous dissection should be performed and minimally invasive techniques must be selected to avoid major complications such as bleeding, iatrojenic neurovascular damage etc. Particularly, resection of the posterior longitudinal ligament must be a little wider then standart discectomy procedure for placing intervertebral implants or grafts. During this procedure, retraction of the dura and roots must be gentle and care. While replacing the implant, surgeon should use scopy for right and exact position and level of it.

6. Conclusion

As a conclusion, anatomical knowledge of the vertebral column and/or spinal cord and also careful preoperative evaluation of the cases as both clinically and radiologically are of importance for realizing successful approach on the degenerative disc diseases.

7. References

Albert T.J., Eichenbaum M.D. (2004) Goals of cervical disc replacement. *Spine J* 4:292S–293S

Aldskogius, H., Arvidsson, J. & Grant, G. (1985) The reaction of primary sensory neurons to peripheral nerve injury with particular emphasis on transganglionic changes. *Brain Res* 357(1): 27-46.

April, E.W. (1990) Clinical anatomy. *The National Medical Series for Independent Study*. 2nd ed. Harwal Publishing Company, USA.

Aryan H.E., Newman C.B., Gold J.J., Acosta Jr F.L., Coover C, Ames C.P. (2008) Percutaneous Axial Lumbar Interbody Fusion (AxiaLIF) of the L5-S1 Segment: Initial Clinical and Radiographic Experience. Minim Invas Neurosurg 51: 225– 230)

Ashkenazi E., Smorgick Y., Rand N., Millgram M.A., Mirovsky Y., Floman Y. (2005) Anterior decompression combined with corpectomies and discectomies in the management of multilevel cervical myelopathy: a hybrid decompression and fixation technique. *J Neurosurg Spine* 3: 205–209

Bao Q.B., Yuan H.A. (2002) New technologies in spine: nucleus replacement. *Spine* 27: 1245–1247

Bao Q.B., Yuan H.A. (2002) Prosthetic disc replacement: the future? *Clin Orthop* 394:139–145

Bao Q.B., Songer M., Pimenta L., Werner D., Reyes-Sanchez A.,Balsano M., Agrillo U., Coric D., Davenport K., Yuan H. (2007) Nubac disc artyhroplasty: preclinical studies and preliminary safety and efficacy evaluations. *SAS J* 1: 36–45

Battie M.G., Videman T., Parent E. (2004) Lumbar disc degeneration: epidemiology and genetics influences. *Spine* 29: 2679–2690

Benglis D.M., Vanni S., Levi A.D. (2009) An anatomical study of the lumbosacral plexus as related to thr minimally invasive transpsoas approach to the lumbar spine. *Neurosurg Spine.* 10(2):139-44.

Benglis D., Elhammady S., Levi A., Vanni S.(2008) Minimally invasive anterolateral approaches for the treatment of back pain and adult degenerative deformity. *Neurosurgery* 68: 191–196

Bergey D.L., Villavicencio A.T., Goldstein T., Regan J.J.(2004) Endoscopic lateral transpsoas approach to the lumbar spine. *Spine* 29: 1681–1688

Bertagnoli R., Vazquez R.J. (2003) The anterolateral transpsoatic approach (ALPA). A new technique for implanting prosthetic disc nucleus devices. *J Spinal Disord* 16: 398-404

Blume H.G., Rojas C.H. (1981) Unilateral lumbar interbody fusion (posterior approach)utilizing dowel graft. *J Neurol Orthop Surg* 2: 171-175.

Bono C.M., Vaccaro A.R. (2007) Interspinous process devices in the lumbar spine. *J Spinal Disord Tech.* 20(3): 255–261

Boyd L.M., Carter A.J. (2006) Injectable biomaterials and vertebral endplate treatment for repair and regeneration of the intervertebral disc. *Eur Spine J* 15(Suppl 3): 414–421

Bryan V.E. (2002) Cervical motion segment replacement. *Eur Spine J* 11(Suppl 2): 92–97

Buric J.,Pulidori M. (2011) Long-term reduction in pain and disability after surgery with the interspinous device for intervertebral assisted motion (DIAM) spinal stabilization system in patients with low back pain: 4-year follow-up from a longitudinal prospective case series. Josip Buric *Eur Spine J* DOI 10.1007/s00586-011-1697-6)

Butt M.F., Farooq M., Dhar S.A., Mir M.R., Mir B.A., Kangoo K.A. (2007) Retrospective analysis of the occurrence of radiologically detectable surgical error in cases of failed pedicle screw implants. *Acta Orthop Belg.* 73(4): 500-6.

Chaichana K.L., Mukherjee D., Adogwa O., Cheng J.S., McGirt M.J. (2011) Correlation of preoperative depression and somatic perception scales with postoperative disability and quality of life after lumbar discectomy. J Neurosurg Spine. Feb;14(2): 261-7.

Chen B.L.,Wei F.X., Ueyama K., Xie D.H., Sannohe A., Liu S.Y.(2011) Adjacent segment degeneration after single-segment PLIF: the risk factor for degeneration and its impact on clinical outcomes. *Eur Spine J* DOI 10.1007/s00586-011-1888-1

Cevei M., Roşca E., Liviu L., Muţiu G., Stoicănescu D., Vasile L. (2011) Imagistic and histopathologic concordances in degenerative lesions of intervertebral disks. *Rom J Morphol Embryol.* 52(1 Suppl):327-32.

Cloward R.B. (1953)The treatment of ruptured lumbar intervertebral discs by vertebral body fusion: indications, operating technique, after care. *J Neurosurg* 10: 154-168.

Cloyd J.M., Malhotra N.R., Weng L., Chen W., Mauck R.L., Elliott D.M. (2007) Material properties in unconfined compression of human nucleus pulposus, injectable hyaluronic acid-base hydrogels and tissue engineering scaffolds. *Eur Spine J* 16(11):1892-8. Epub 2007 Jul 28.

Costa F.,Sassi M., Ortolina A.,Cardia A., Assietti R., Zerbi A., Lorenzetti M.,Galbusera F., Fornari M. (2011) Stand-alone cage for posterior lumbar interbody fusion in the treatment of high-degree degenerative disc disease: design of a new device for an "old" technique. A prospective study on a series of 116 patients. *Eur Spine J* (2011) 20 (Suppl 1):S46–S56

Cox C.S., Rodgers W.B., Gerber E.J. (2008) XLIF in the treatment of single-level lumbar spondylolisthesis: 6 month and 1 year follow up. *J Neurosurg* 108:A853, 2008 (Abstract)

Cummings, C.W., Fredrickson, J.M., Harker, L.A., Krause, C.J., & Schuller, D.E. (1993). *Otolaryngology-Head and Neck Surgery.* 2nd ed. Vol I, Mosby Year Book.

de Maat G.,Puntl.M., van Rhijn L.W., Schurink G.H.,van Ooij A. (2009) Removal of the Charite´ Lumbar Artificial Disc Prosthesis Surgical Technique. *J Spinal Disord Tech* 22; 5:334-339

Derby R., Howard M.W., Grant J.M., Lettice J.J., Van Peteghem P.K., Ryan D.P. (1999) The ability of pressurecontrolled discography to predict surgical and nonsurgical outcomes. *Spine* 24: 364-372.

Dezawa A., Yamane T., Mikami H., Miki H. (2000) Retroperitoneal laparoscopic lateral approach to the lumbar spine. *J Spinal Disord* 13: 138–143

Di Martino A., Vaccaro A.R., Lee J.Y., Denaro V., Lim M.R. (2005) Nucleus pulposus replacement: basic science and indications for clinical use. *Spine* 30: 16– 22

Ebraheim N.A., Xu R., Darwich M., Yeasting R.A. (1997) Anatomic relations between the lumbar pedicle and the adjacent neural structures. *Spine* (Phila Pa 1976). 15; 22(20):2338-41.

Edeland H.G. (1981) Suggestions for a total elasto-dynamic intervertebral disc prosthesis. *Biomater Med Devices Artif Organs.* 9(1):65-72.

Enker P., Steffee A., Mcmillan C., Keppler L., Biscup R., Miller S. (1993) Artificial disc replacement. Preliminary report with a 3-year minimum follow-up. *Spine* 18:1061-1070

Fekete T.F., Porchet F. (2010) Overview of disc arthroplasty-past, present and future. *Acta Neurochir (Wien).* 152(3):393-404. Review.

Fernstrom U. (1966) Arthroplasty with intercorporal endoprothesis in herniated disc and in painful disc. *Acta Chir Scand* (Suppl) 357:154–159

Ferrera, P.C., & Chandler, R. (1994) Anesthesia in the emergency setting: Part II. Head and neck, eye and rib injuries. *Am Fam Physician* 15; 50(4):797-800.

Gloria A., Borzacchiello A., Causa F., Ambrosio L. (2010) Rheological Characterization of Hyaluronic Acid Derivatives as Injectable Materials Toward Nucleus Pulposus Regeneration. *J Biomater Appl.* [Epub ahead of print]

Gocmen-Mas N., Karabekir H., Ertekin T., Senan S., Edizer M., Yazici C., Duyar I. (2010) Evaluation of Lumbar Vertebral Body and Disc: A Stereological Morphometric Study. *Int. J. Morphol.,* 28(3):841-847.

Gornet M.F., Burkus J.K., Dryer R.F., Peloza J.H. (2011) Lumbar Disc Arthroplasty with MAVERICK™ Disc Versus Stand-Alone Interbody Fusion: A Prospective,Randomized, Controlled, Multicenter Investigational Device Exemption Trial. *Spine (Phila Pa 1976).* [Epub ahead of print]

Haghighat, K. (2007). "Bone augmentation techniques."*J Periodontol* 78(3): 377-96.

Harms J.(1997) True spondylolisthesis reduction and more segmental fusion in spondylolisthesis. In: Bridwell KH, DeWald RL (Eds.). *The Textbook of Spinal Surgery.* 2nd Ed. Philadelphia, Lippincott-Raven.

Hedman T.P., Kostuik J.P., Fernie G.R., Hellier W.G. (1991) Design of an intervertebral disc prosthesis. *Spine* 16(Suppl 6):256–260

Hilibrand A.S., Robbins M. (2004) Adjacent segment degeneration and adjacent segment disease: the consequences of spinal fusion? *Spine J* 4: 190–194

Hioki A., Miyamoto K., Hosoe H., Sugiyama S., Suzuki N., Shimizu K. (2011) Cantilever transforaminal lumbar interbody fusion for upper lumbar degenerative diseases (minimum 2 years follow up). *Yonsei Med J.* 52(2): 314-21.

Hutton M.J., Bayer J.H., Powell J., Sharp D.J. (2011) Modic vertebral body changes: The natural history as assessed by consecutive magnetic resonance imaging. *Spine* (Phila Pa 1976). Feb 25. [Epub ahead of print]

Joshi A., Mehta S., Vresilovic E., Karduna A., Marcolongo M. (2005) Nucleus implant parameters significantly change the compressive stiffness of the human lumbar intervertebral disc. *J Biomech Eng* 127: 536–540

Junjie D., Mo L., Hao L., Hao M., Qizhen H., Zhuojing L. (2011) Early follow-up outcomes after treatment of degenerative disc disease with the discover cervical disc prosthesis *The Spine Journal* 11: 281–289

Kabir S.M., Gupta S.R., Casey A.T. (2010) Lumbar interspinous spacers: a systematic review of clinical and biomechanical evidence. *Spine* (Phila Pa 1976). 1; 35(25): 1499-506.

Kaiser M.G., Haid R.W.Jr., Subach B.R., Barnes B., Rodts G.E.Jr. (2002) Anterior cervical plating enhances arthrodesis after discectomy and fusion with cortical allograft. *Neurosurgery* 50: 229-238

Karabekir H.S., Atar E.K., Yaycioglu S., Yildizhan A.(2008) Comparison of unilateral posterior lumbar interbody fusion and bilateral posterior lumbar interbody fusion with simple discectomy at degenerative disc herniations. *Neurosciences* 13 (3): 248-252

Karabekir H.S., Korkmaz S., Ozturk U. (2009) Comparison of unilateral posterior lumbar interbody fusion with simple discectomy at degenerative disc disease. *The J Turkish Spinal Surgery* 20 (1): 47- 52.

Karabekir H.S., Yildizhan A.,Atar K.E., Yaycioglu S., Gocmen-Mas N., Yazici C. (2010) Effect of ligamenta flava hypertrophy on lumbar disc herniation with contralateral symptoms and signs: a clinical and morphometric study. *Arch Med Sci* 6(4): 617-622

Karabekir H.S.,Mas N.G., Edizer M.,Ertekin T., Yazici C, Atamturk D (2011). Lumbar Vertebra Morphometry and Stereological Assesment of Intervertebral Space Volumetry: A Methodological Study *Ann Anatomy* 193(3): 231-6. Epub 2011 Apr 2.

Klara P.M., Ray C.D. (2002) Artificial nucleus replacement: clinical experience. *Spine* 27:1374-1377

Kostuik J.P. (1997) Intervertebral disc replacement. In: Bridwell KH, DeWald RL (eds) *The textbook of spinal surgery*, 2nd edn. Lippincott-Raven, Philadelphia.

Krumlauf R. (1994) Hox genes in vertebrate development. *Cell.* 29; 78(2): 191-201. Review.

Kumar M.N., Jacquot F., Hall H. (2001) Long-term follow-up of functional outcomes and radiographic changes at adjacent levels following lumbar spine fusion for degenerative disc disease. *Eur Spine J* 10: 309-313

Kuslich S.D., Ulstrom C.L., Griffith S.L., Ahern J.W., Dowdle J.D. (1998) The Bagby and Kuslich method of lumbar interbody fusion. History, techniques, and 2-year follow-up results of a United States prospective, multicenter trial. *Spine* 23: 1267-1279

Lafuente J., Casey A.T., Petzold A., Brew S. (2005) The Bryan cervical disc prosthesis a san alternative to arthrodesis in the treatment of cervical spondylosis. *J Bone Joint Surg Br* 87(4): 508-512

Larson J.W., Chadderon R.C., Georgescu H., Lee D., Hubert M., Werkmeister-Lewis L., Irrang J.,Gilbertson L.G., Kang J.D. (2006) Prevention of intervertebral disc degeneration after surgical discectomy using an injectable nucleus pulposus prosthesis. In: *Proceedings of the 52nd annual meeting of the orthopaedic research society, Chicago, USA.*

Lee C.K. (1988) Accelerated degeneration of the segment adjacent to a lumbar fusion. *Spine* 13: 375-377

Lee C.K., Langrana N.A., Parsons J.R., Zimmerman M.C. (1991) Development of a prosthetic intervertebral disc. *Spine* 16(Suppl 6): 253-255

Lee C.S., Hwang C.J., Lee S.W., Ahn Y.J., Kim Y.T., Lee D.H., Lee M.Y. (2009) Risk factors for adjacent segment disease after lumbar fusion. *Eur Spine J* 11: 1637-1643

Lin P., Cautilli R., Joyce M. (1983) Posterior lumbar interbody fusion. *Clin Orthop* 180: 154-167.

Lipetz J.S. (2002) Pathophysiology of inflammatory, degenerative, and compressive radiculopathies. *Phys Med Rehabil Clin N Am.* 13(3): 439-49. Review.

Lundborg, G. (1988) Intraneural microcirculation. *Orthop Clin North Am* 19(1): 1-12.Review.

Mallo M., Vinagre T., Carapuço M. (2009) The road to the vertebral formula. *Int J Dev Biol.* 53(8-10): 1469-81. Review.

Marks R.C., Houston T., Thulbourne T. (1992) Facet joint injection and facet nerve block: a randomised comparison in 86 patients with chronic low back pain. *Pain* 49: 325-328

Matz P.G., Pritchard P.R., Hadley M.N. (2007) Anterior cervical approach for the treatment of cervical myelopathy. *Neurosurgery* 60(Suppl): 64–70

Mayer H.M. (1997) A new microsurgical technique for minimally invasive anterior lumbar interbody fusion. *Spine* 22: 691–699

McAfee P.C., Regan J.J., Geis W.P., Fedder I.L. (1998) Minimally invasive anterior retroperitoneal approach to the lumbar spine Emphasis on the lateral BAK. *Spine* 23: 1476-1484

McAfee P.C., Phillips F.M., Allen T.R., Regan J.J., Albert T.J., Cappuccino A., Devine J.G., Ahrens J.E., Hipp J.A. (2009) Cervical disc replacement in patients with and without previous adjacent level fusion surgery: a prospective study. *Spine* (Phila Pa 1976). 15; 34(6): 556-65.

Moore, K.L. (1992) *Clinically orianted anatomy.* The Williams and Wilkind Company USA.

Mummaneni P.V., Burkus J.K., Haid R.W.,Traynelis V.C., Zdeblick T.A. (2007) Clinical and radiographic analysis of cervical disc arthroplasty compared with allograft fusion: a randomized controlled clinical trial. *J Neurosurg Spine* 6(3): 198–209

Nachemson A.L. (1992) Challenge of the artificial disc. In: Weinstein JN (ed) *Clinical efficacy and outcome in the diagnosis and treatment of low back pain.* Raven Press, New York,USA

Okuda S., Oda T., Miyauchi A., Tamura S., Hashimoto Y., Yamasaki S., Haku T., Kanematsu F., Ariga K., Ohwada T., Aono H., Hosono N., Fuji T., Iwasaki M. (2008) Lamina horizontalization and facet tropism as the risk factors for adjacent segment degeneration after PLIF. *Spine* 33: 2754-2758

Park P., Garton H.J., Gala V.C., Hoff J.T., McGillicuddy J.E. (2004) Adjacent segment disease after lumbar or lumbosacral fusion: review of the literature. *Spine* 29: 1938-1944

Patel K.P.,Sandy J.D., Akeda K., Miyamoto K., Chujo T., An H.S., Masuda K. (2007) Aggrecanases and aggrecanasegenerated fragments in the human intervertebral disc at early and advanced stages of disc degeneration, *Spine* (Phil Pa 1976) 32 (23) : 2596-2603.

Pimenta L., McAfee .PC., Cappuccino A., Bellera F.P., Link H.D. (2007) Superiority of multilevel cervical arthroplasty outcomes versus single-level outcomes: 229 consecutive PCM prostheses. *Spine* 32(12): 1337-1344

Ray C.D. (1997) Threaded titanium cages for lumbar intebody fusions. *Spine* 22(6): 67-80.

Rahm M.D., Hall B.H. (1996) Adjacent-segment degeneration after lumbar fusion with instrumentation: a retrospective study. *J Spinal Disord* 9: 392-400

Rothman R.H., Simeone F.A., Bernini P.M. (1982) Lumbar disc disease. In: Rothman RH, Simeone FA (eds) The spine, 2nd edn. WB Saunders, Philadelphia, USA

Schwarzer A.C., Aprill C.N., Derby R., Fortin J., Kine G., Bogduk N. (1994) Clinical features of patients with pain stemming from the lumbar zygapophysial joints. Is the lumbar facet syndrome a clinical entity? *Spine* (Phila Pa 1976) 19:1132-1137

Schwarzer A.C., Aprill C.N., Derby R., Fortin J., Kine G., Bogduk N. (1994) The false-positive rate of uncontrolled diagnostic blocks of the lumbar zygapophysial joints. *Pain* 58:195–200

Sekhon L.H.S. (2004) Cervical arthroplasty in the management of spondylotic myelopathy: 18-month results. *Neurosurg Focus* 17(3): 55–61

Sekhon L.H.S. (2004) Two-level artificial disc placement for spondylotic cervical myelopathy. *J Clin Neurosci* 11(4): 412–415

Snell R.S. (2011) *Clinical Anatomy*. Williams and Wilkins 8th ed.Walters Kluwer, USA.

Standring S., Ellis H., Healy J.C., Johnson D., Williams A., Collins P. (2005) *Gray's Anatomy* (ed 39). London, Churchill Livingstone.

Steffee A., Sitkowski D.(1988) Posterior lumbar interbody fusion and plates. *Clin Orthop* 227: 99-102.

Sunderland S., (1951) A Classification of Peripheral Nerve Injuries Producing Loss of Function *Brain* 74(4): 491-516.

Taner D. (2004) Functional Neuroanatomy. 4th ed. ODTU Press, Ankara, Turkey.

Turner J.A., Ersek M., Herron L., Haselkorn J., Kent D., Ciol M.A., Deyo R. (1992) Patientoutcomes after lumbar spinal fusions. *JAMA* 268: 907–911.

Turner J.A., Herron L., Deyo R.A. (1993) Meta-analysis of the results of lumbar spine fusion. *Acta Orthop Scand Suppl* 251: 120–122

Van de Graaff. (1998). *Human Anatomy 5th ed*. WBC McGraw-Hill Companies, USA.

Van Zundert J., Huntoon M., Patijn J., Lataster A., Mekhail N., van Kleef M. (2010) Cervical radicular pain. *Pain Practice.Pain Pract.* 10(1): 1-17. Review.

Waddell G., Gibson J.N.A., Grant I. (2000) Surgical treatment of lumbar disc prolapse and degenerative lumbar disc disease. In: Nachemson AL, Jonssom E (eds) *Neck and back pain*. Lippincott Williams & Wilkins, Philadelphia.

Weatherly C.R., Prickett C.F., O.Brien J.P.(1986) Discogenic pain persisting despite solid posterior fusion. *J Bone Joint Surg* 68-B:142-143.

Weinstein J.N. (ed) (1992) *Clinical efficacy and outcome in the diagnosis and treatment of low back pain*. Raven Press, New York

Wellik D.M. (2007) Hox patterning of the vertebrate axial skeleton. *Dev Dyn.* 236(9): 2454-2463 Review.

West W., West K.P., Younger E.N., Cornwall D. (2010) Degenerative disc disease of the lumbar spine on MRI. *West Indian Med J.* 59(2): 192-5.

Wiggins G.C., Shaffrey C.I. (2007) Dorsal surgery for myelopathy and myeloradiculopathy. *Neurosurgery* 60(Suppl): 71–81

Williams P.L., Bannister L.H., Berry M.M., Patricia C.,Dyson M., Dussek J.E., Ferguson M.W.J. (1995) *Gray's Anatomy*. 38th ed. Churchill-Livingstone, UK.

Winn H.R. (2004) *Youmans Neurological Surgery*. 5th ed. Saunders, Philadelphia,PA., USA.

Woodburne R.T., Burkel W.E. (1994) *Essentials of Human Anatomy* 9th ed New York, Oxford University Press.

Zencica P., Chaloupka R., Hladı́ková J., Krbec M. (2010) Adjacent segment degeneration after lumbosacral fusion in spondylolisthesis: a retrospective radiological and clinical analysis. *Acta Chir Orthop Traumatol Cech* 77: 124–130

Section 2

Functional Neurosurgery

4

Targeting the Subthalamic Nucleus for Deep Brain Stimulation in Parkinson Disease: The Impact of High Field Strength MRI

Dirk Winkler, Marc Tittgemeyer, Karl Strecker, Axel Goldammer,
Jochen Helm, Johannes Schwarz and Jürgen Meixensberger
Department of Neurosurgery, University of Leipzig, Leipzig
Germany

1. Introduction

Functional neurosurgery is the only surgical alternative treatment for patients with Parkinson's disease (PD) (Agid, 1999; Benzzouz & Hallett, 2000; Beric et al., 2001; DeLong & Wichmann, 2001; Dowsey-Limousin et al., 2001; Hariz & Fodstad, 2002; Kopper et al., 2003; Krause et al., 2001; Vesper et al., 2002). Dopamine deficiency in Parkinson's disease leads to increased neuronal activity. Regulation of this overactivity using electrical stimulation of the basal ganglia (deep brain stimulation – DBS) has become an attractive neurosurgical option of alternative treatment strategy (Limousin et al., 1998; Kupsch & Earl, 1999). The subthalamic nucleus (STN) is the key structure for motor control through the basal ganglia and is mostly used as stimulation target since here, all cardinal symptoms of PD can be effectively ameliorated (Anderson et al., 2005; Benabid et al., 1998; Dujardin et al, 2001; Limousin et al., 1998; Martinez-Martin et al., 2002; Koller et al., 2001; Krack et al., 1998; Lopiano et al., 2001; Volkmann et al., 2001). Possible mechanisms of DBS include depolarization blockade, release of local inhibitory neurotransmitters, antidromic activation of inhibitory neurons, and jamming of abnormal neuronal firing patterns. The clinical experiences and practice confirm the beneficial effect of chronic bilateral STN-DBS.

Especially the definition of the target area as well as positioning of test and permanent electrodes are subjects of ongoing debates, reflecting the different possibilities, including ventriculography, CT-guidance, MR-imaging and combined techniques (Hariz & Bergenheim, 1990, 1993). Advances in image acquisition, image postprocessing as well as potentials of multimodality including image supported surgery, microelectrode-recording (MER) and macrostimulation technologies have been the driving forces behind the resurgence in the use of functional stereotaxic surgery. Besides the precise selection of Parkinson patients, which are ideal candidates for deep brain stimulation, correct preoperative target definition and intraoperative target localization are the most important factors for surgical success and good clinical outcome (Lopiano et al., 2002).

This is the first comparative study, which evaluates the value of 3 Tesla MRI data for the definition of the STN as the target region for deep brain stimulation in patients with PD. This study shows the results of DBS-electrode placement using different MR-imaging (T1w,

T2w; 1,5T, 3T), which were used for preoperative visualization of the target region and anatomical landmarks as the precondition for the definition of target coordinates. In the next step, we systematically investigated the effects of bilateral STN-DBS on motor functions and medication in both groups in a twelve-month follow up.

2. Methods

The described prospective study included 27 patients (20 male, 7 female) with idiopathic PD in whom STN-DBS surgery was realized. Patient age ranges from 39-75 years. The mean age of males and females was 62.9 years. The mean duration of the disease was 12.3 years, ranging from 4 to 17 years.

Patients qualified for stereotaxic and functional neurosurgery, showed no evidence for psychiatric illness, cognitive impairment, severe brain atrophy, or other substantial medical problems of laboratory abnormalities, dementia, major focal or severe diffuse brain abnormalities, extensive brain atrophy nor any severe systemic internal disease, which could exclude stimulation therapy.

For targeting procedure image fusion of preoperative acquired 3D T1w and T2w 1.5T MR-image series ("Intera", Philips, Germany, 13 patients, group I) and 3D T1w 1.5 T and T2w 3 T MR-image series (Bruker, Germany, 14 patients, group II) was used and the possible benefit of 3 T MRI was evaluated, analyzing surgical and clinical data. In all cases with PD we preferred a bilateral electrode insertion in a single session, beginning with the more symptomatic side. Direct magnetic resonance imaging-based anatomic targeting was used.

2.1 Image acquisition and planning procedure

At present time a wide variety of target localization and implantation techniques exists (Limousin et al., 1998; Kupsch & Earl, 1999). Traditional stereotaxic algorithm has been based on an externally fixed stereotaxic frame that encompasses the patient's head and upon which the micromanipulating equipment can be mounted and maneuvered with highest accuracy (Dujardin et al., 2001; Martinez-Martin, 2002). Corresponding to the existing stereotactic frames and their refinements, all stereotaxic frames have been optimized to allow nearly artefact-free image data sets and to guarantee a precise and reproducible definition of target and entry points. Typically, these frames are mounted on the day of surgery, just before acquisition of planning image data sets.

Beginning this step of functional neurosurgery the patient is free of any L-Dopa medication as a precondition for macrostimulation and awake-neurological examination. Consequently, tremor-related motion artefacts during image acquisition are encountered, despite of the patient's head fixation using headholders (CT) and headcoils (MRI), which reduce the accuracy of image co-registration theoretically and possible practically. Nevertheless, the delay involved with frame fixation, image acquisition, planning and three dimensional checking can take several hours depending on personal and institutional experiences and the patient's properties as a kind of stress just before surgery.

In our study on the day of surgery the patient's head was fixed in an MR-compatible ceramic head holder (Zamorano-Dujovny, ZD, Fa. Stryker, Howmedica, Leibinger, Germany) in local anaesthesia. Position of the head ring was chosen in such a way that pin

Targeting the Subthalamic Nucleus for Deep Brain Stimulation in Parkinson Disease: The Impact of High Field
Strength MRI

69

placement and expected metal artefacts of the screw tips were away from the axial plane of the target point (STN) and any structures of interest.

For functional and surgical planning it is necessary to map points and regions of interest from one patient image to another that has been taken at a different time or/and with a different image method. In this study the combination of T1w and T2w image series seemed to be the most practical way. The rational behind this procedure is that T2w image data allow an excellent visualization of target structures (STN) and neighbouring anatomical landmarks (Nc. ruber). The T1w images are used for stereotaxic planning and realization of surgery.

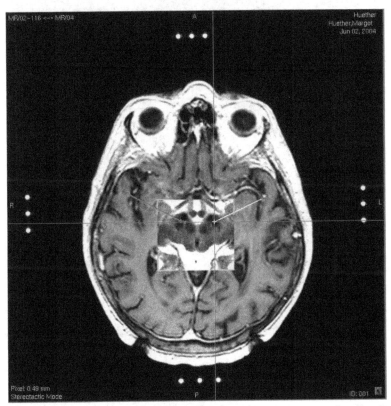

Fig. 1. Postprocessing result (image fusion) for following definition of target coordinates basing of 3D T1w and T2w MR image data of the region of interest (T1w 1.5 T MRI and T2w 3 T MRI)

Corresponding to the different possibilities we analysed two patient cohorts: in the first group (group I) 1.5 Tesla T1w (3D-magnetization-prepared rapid gradient echo-TE 4,6 msec, TR 25 msec) and T2w (Turbo spin echo-TE 120 msec, TR 4389 msec) image series with the following parameters: matrix 256 x 256, slice thickness: 1 mm ("Intera", Philips, Germany, 1.5 Tesla) were acquired and fused together slice identically (Fig. 1). In group II the 1.5 Tesla T1w image series ("Intera", Philips, Germany, 1.5 Tesla) was combined and fused with the

T2w image series, acquired in the 3 Tesla Bruker MRI (matrix 256 x 256, slice thickness: 1 mm, Turbo spin echo-TE 355 msec, TR 3500 msec), Max-Planck-Institute of Cognition and Neuroscience, Leipzig, Germany. Just before magnetic resonance image acquisition (T1w MRI) contrast media was given in both groups in a standard dose (0.1 mmol/kg bodyweight Gd-DTPA, Magnevist, Schering, Germany) to improve detail informations as well as to identify passing vessels.

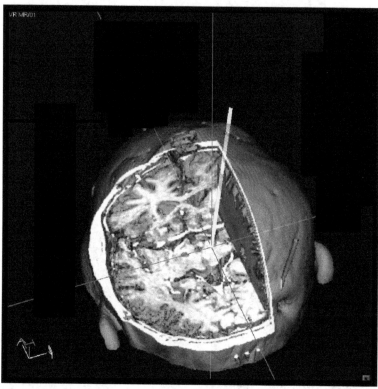

Fig. 2. Virtual 3D reconstruction of planned electrode trajectory

Stereotaxic coordinates were calculated with the "Remote surgical planning software" (RSPS, Fa. Stryker, Howmedica, Leibinger, Germany) or with the VoXim® / microTargeting™ , IVS Technology, Germany, FHC, USA. In the following steps, image postprocessing, definition of functional, entry and target coordinates and visualization of planed trajectories take place. In general, the final stage in the presurgical planning process involves reviewing the proposed trajectory interactively in the sagittal, axial and coronal plane and checking the coordinates verified that the cannula passes exactly to the defined target point. The surgical planning process involved the identification and adaptation of the target using the typical appearance of the STN and the Nc. ruber in T2w image series and reviewing the proposed trajectory interactively in the sagittal, axial and coronal plane. Any field inhomogeneities of the used MRI could be ruled out in previous studies (Figure 3).

Entry and target points were chosen and the coordinates of the space were calculated
automatically by the special „frame-based stereotaxy" software program, including the A, B,
C, D and E values for the target device of the stereotaxic system. These coordinates were the
base for the intraoperative used target arc system, which was connected with the stereotaxic
head ring (Zamorano-Dujovny, ZD, Leibinger, Germany). A phantom system called target
point simulator was used for intraoperative control of coordinates. Checking the coordinates
verified that the cannula passes exactly to the defined target point.

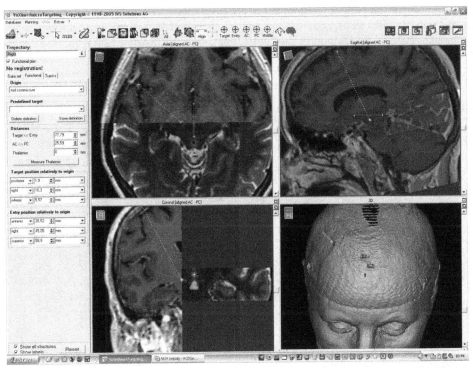

Fig. 3. Identification and adaptation of the target-coordinates using the sagital, axial and
coronal plane.

2.2 Functional neurosurgery

In the surgical part, the mild sedated patient was transferred to the operating theatre
without a possibility of frame dislocation and was fixed normally using a special adapter
unit. In the operating theatre patients was lying in a 45° upright position and was mild
sedated with intermittend injections of midazolam to allow motor and verbal testing during
intraoperative testing stimulation.

Head was cleaned and draped with the entry site in view. Under local anaesthesia and mild
sedation, a burr hole craniotomy was made at the desirable entry point and the target arch
was installed. The burr hole was placed in the standard location near the coronal suture and
approximately 3 to 5 cm from the midline. Five stainless-steel microelectrodes were inserted
stereotaxically using multi-channel microelectrodes (Leadpoint 4, medtronic, USA).

Microrecording was performed to identify the STN signature (frequency, pattern, amplitude) as a reliable criterion for the correct electrode position. Target signals were analysed for defining STN target, including frequency, firing rates and interspike intervals (Hutchison et al., 1998, Raeva et al., 1991, 1993).

Recording was started 10 mm above the target and was continued to 4 mm below the supposed STN. The target for the final placement of the electrode was confirmed by macrostimulation using the microelectrode housing cannula. The target was confirmed by the responses of the patient to stimuli (130 Hz frequency, 0-5.0 mA stimulation amplitude, 60 sec pulse width) delivered through the macroelectrode. During test stimulation eye movement, speech, contraction of the contralateral face, neck, tongue, skeletal muscle, and the suppression of tremor and rigidity were checked. Mostly, clinical testing indicating a dramatic improvement of tremor, akinesis and rigidity of the contralateral limb and showed a disappearance of drug-induced dyskinesia postoperatively (Figure 4)

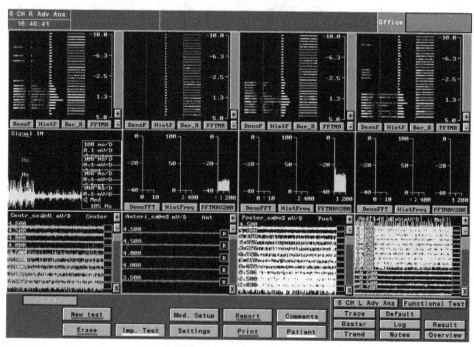

Fig. 4. Microelectrode – recoding for visualization of typical STN-signature along the z-axis

Final positioning of the permanent electrode (DBS electrode, model 3389, Medtronic, USA) was monitored on the fluoroscopy screen to avoid discrepancies between planned and real localization of the tip of the electrode. After electrode positioning the electrode was secured to the patient's skull using bone cement and miniplates for fixation (Figure 5). The same procedure was repeated on the other side. After all neurosurgical steps stereotactic frame was removed from the patient's head and implantation of impulse generator (Kinetra Impulsgenerator, model 7428, Medtronic, Minneapolis) was done under general anaesthesia.

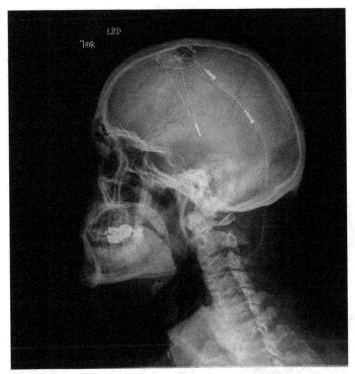

Fig. 5. Real position of the stimulation electrodes, documented by fluoroscopy

On the same or next day patients underwent postoperative MRI to rule out any surgery associated complications (Figure 6a, b). Stimulation testing and wound control took place and depending on their and the family conditions they was discharged home or to rehabilitation. In regular follow-ups, medication was checked and adjustments were made to optimise the stimulation parameters After placement of permanent electrodes, a pulse generator (Kinetra Impulsgenerator, model 7428, Medtronic, Minneapolis) was implanted in the infraclavicular fossa and connected to the electrodes. The following stimulation consisted of continuous square-wave pulses (frequency: 130 Hz, pulse duration: 120 μs, amplitude: 2.5 V). Clinical examination was performed to rule out any postoperative complications, motor, especially oculomotor and speech abnormalities. Postoperative MRI confirmed the electrode position.

2.3 Results

Planning procedure for following STN-DBS using preoperative acquired 1.5T and 3T MRI data is a reliable tool for successful stereotaxic treatment of PD. Using T1w image date after injection of contrast media an excellent visualization of anatomical details (ventricle structures, sulci and gyri) as well as passing vessels could be guaranteed. High resolution 3 Tesla MRI (T2w) allowed brilliant identification of the typical almond-shaped STN and the Nc. rubber with their typical hypointense shape. Image fusion was realized manually using

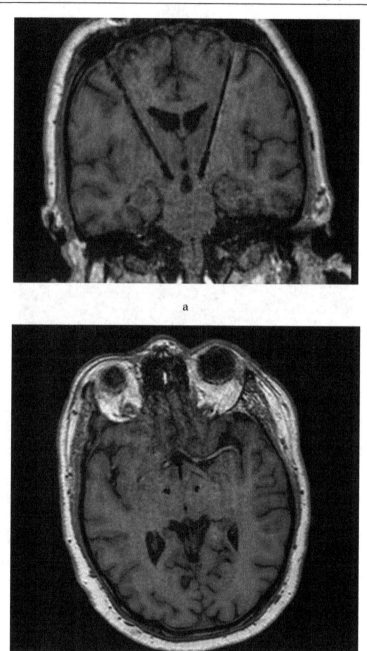

Fig. 6. a, b: Postoperative control of electrode positioning in different planes (a: coronar, b: axial), confirmed by small metal artefacts

anatomical landmarks with an accuracy of 0.9 mm, ranging from 0.4-1.1 mm. Corresponding
to the anatomical markers and the theoretical target coordinates the STN position was
superior to the substantia nigra, lateral to the anterior portion of the red nucleus and medial
to the internal capsule: The longest medial-lateral and ventral-posterior diameter of STN
was aimed and located immediately lateral to the anterior aspect of the Nc. rubber in the
axial plane. With the help of ben gun system five electrodes were implanted simultaneously
in the target region to validate target region electrophysiologically. Typical STN signature,
representing neuronal activity could be documented in implanted microelectrodes. After
microrecording macrostimulation was performed using electrodes with the best STN signal
to confirm correct electrode placement using common stimulation parameter In both groups
the image fusion accuracy was with 0.37 (group I) and 0.40 (group II) nearly the same and
allowed a precise and slice identical correlation of both, T1w and T2w image series in both
modalities (1.5 T, 3 T)(Table 1). The number of microelectrodes which detected a typical STN
signature during MER of both sites increased from 6.7 (group I) to 7.1 (group II) averagely
and showed a tendency of a safer localization of the expected target point basing on
preoperative acquired image data in the second group. Further data of planning (functional
coordinates) and surgical (surgical time) procedures are summarized in Table 1 and
correspond with planning data of other studies (Okun et al., 2005).

radiological and surgical data	Group I (n=13) T1-w (1.5 Tesla) T2-w (1.5 Tesla)	Group II (n=14) T1-w (1.5 Tesla) T2-w (3.0 Tesla)
fusion accuracy, mean (min - max)	0.37 (0.2 – 0.6)	0.40 (0.2 – 0.7)
surgical time (min) mean (min - max)	267 (202 – 313)	247 (160 – 302)
functional coordinates x y z	± 11.25 - 1.95 - 4.15	± 10.4 - 2.05 - 4.45
active electrodes, mean (min - max)	6.7 (2 – 9)	7.1 (4 – 9)

Table 1. Summarized radiological, planning and surgical data

As a result of this, the functional coordinates have the biggest differences in the x-coordinates,
but were comparable in the others. Interestingly, in group I the central track (48%) dominated
as the best traject for the placement of the permanent stimulation electrode, which is followed
by the medial one's (20%)(Figure 7). Contrary to this, in group II predominated the anterior
track with 41.7%, compared to 37% of the central track (Figure 8).

In the comparison of both groups we found a domination of the central (group I) and
anterior and central position of the active electrode (group II, Figure 9).

In the postoperative course the mean administered dose of L-dopa decreased significantly in
group I from 698.1 mg/day to 200.0 mg/day twelve months later, that means 28.7 % of the
initial mean dosage and in group II from 686.5 mg/day to 183.3 mg/day (24.9%)(Table 2,

Figure 10). The reduction of L-dopa dose one, two, three and twelve months postoperatively differed not significantly between both groups.

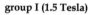

group I (1.5 Tesla)

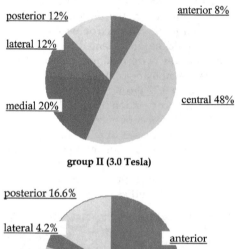

Fig. 8. Distribution of active electrodes in group II (3 Tesla MRI)

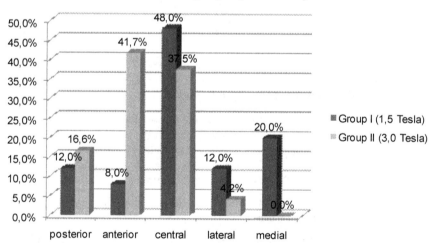

Fig. 9. Distribution of "active" electrodes with typical STN signature, detected by microrecording

L-dopa (daily dose, mg-values given as mean)	Group I (n=13) T1-w (1.5 Tesla) T2-w (1.5 Tesla)	Group II (n=14) T1-w (1.5 Tesla) T2-w (3.0 Tesla)
Preoperative	698.1 SD ± 251	686.5 SD ± 469
Postoperative - one month	170.8 SD ± 151**	170.8 SD ± 123**
Postoperative - two months	112.5 SD ± 210**	187.5 SD ± 131**
Postoperative - three months	155.5 SD ± 212**	212.5 SD ± 75**
Postoperative - twelve months	200.0 SD ± 115**	183.3 SD ± 177**

Table 2. Comparison of preoperative and postoperative L-dopa-medication in both groups. In spite of some irregularities in the course of twelve months the final dose reduction in both groups is comparable and no criteria for the used image modality. (** p < 0.01)

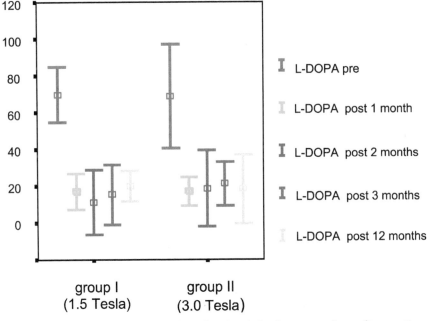

Fig. 10. Pre- and postoperative L-DOPA medication in both groups, depending on time course (preoperative, one, two, three and twelve months after STN-DBS)

The motor ratings improved significantly (p ≤ 0.01) from the preoperative (medication-off) to the stimulator-on (medication-on) conditions in both groups (Table 3, Figure 11). Mean improvement were 70.4% (group I) and 55.4% (group II), respectively, for UPDRS, part III (Table 3, Figure 11). No significant differences between the two groups were seen.

UPDRS (III)	Group I (n=13) T1-w (1.5 Tesla) T2-w (1.5 Tesla)	Group II (n=14) T1-w (1.5 Tesla) T2-w (3.0 Tesla)
Preoperative	43.9 SD ± 20.0	42.6 SD ± 10.0
Postoperative - one month	13.4 SD ± 10.0**	13.6 SD ± 6.2**
Postoperative - twelve months	13.0 SD ± 6.3**	19.0 SD ± 4.5**

(** p < 0.01)

Table 3. Improvement of UPDRS (part III) in both groups up to one year after functional neurosurgery.

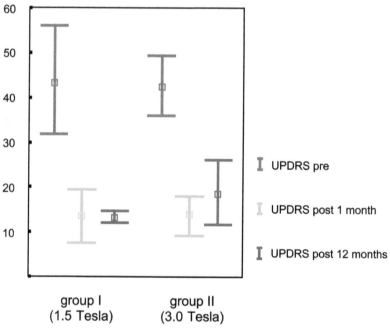

Fig. 11. Clinical effect (UPDRS (part III) up to one year after deep brain stimulation

3. Discussion

The principle of stereotaxic surgery was created by Horsley and Clarke as well as Spiegel, Wycis and Leksell. Stereotaxic surgery is a well established and accurate method and offers increasing possibilities for diagnosis and therapy. Today, stereotaxic localization based on

CT and MRI data is mostly used to guide the neurosurgeon during biopsy and functional neurosurgery with an accuracy of less than one millimetre, which is an essential advantage of used high precision stereotaxic frames. Former studies confirmed the high accuracy of stereotaxic devices despite system associated errors.

The beneficial effect of bilateral STN stimulation for neurosurgical treatment of PD is confirmed by countless studies and groups and should not be the focus of this article. At present time many neurosurgical concepts exist making the functional neurosurgery for PD via STN-DBS safe for patients and surgeons as well. The clinical results with traditional ventriculography, CT-guidance, MR-imaging and combined techniques are comparable. In this STN-DBS study for treatment of idiopathic PD we performed microrecording and macrostimulation as routinely used steps during the stereotaxic procedure, but practiced different MR planning modalities for electrode placement : 1.5 and 3 Tesla MR (T1w and T2w). Differences in both techniques and both groups as well as clinical and surgical data are the initial points for the following discussion.

In this study we used different MR modalities to define the target point and used MER and macrostimulation for electrophysiological respectively clinical validation of chosen trajectories for final electrodes.

The great appeal of 3T MRI is the improvement in image quality and an increased signal-to-noise ratio (SNR). Many are excited about the opportunity to not only use the increased SNR for clearer images, but also the chance to exchange it better resolution and contrast - a fact already well known from comparisons of images obtained at 0.5T, 1T, and 1.5T MRI. In the case of 3T MRI the SNR correlates in approximately linear fashion with field strength, it is roughly twice as great at 3T as at 1.5T. The magnetic susceptibility is exacerbated and the time necessary to acquire satisfactory images can be substantially reduced and motion artifacts can be minimized. Among other benefits, higher contrast may permit reduction of gadolinium doses and, in some cases, earlier detection of disease, a possible stimulus to use higher field systems. These possibilities makes the 3T MRI attractive especially for brain imaging.

Nevertheless, significant obstacles to 3T MRI presented by the physics at higher field strengths. 1. especially the T1 relaxation times are prolonged with increasing magnet field strength, the chemical shift is larger and the susceptibility is stronger. 2. There are safety concerns. The energy deposited in the patient's tissues is fourfold higher at 3T than at 1.5T. Especially with the use of fast spin echo and fluid attenuation inversion recovery (FLAIR), the limit on the specific absorption rate (SAR) power deposition prescribed by the FDA can easily be reached compared to 1.5T MR protocols. Scanner manufacturers are incorporating modified pulse sequences to avoid this problem, which can also be solved by restricting the volume of tissue that is studied in detail.

In our study we couldn´t observe, that the application of 3T MRI could avoid multiple passes of microelectrodes for electrophysiologic confirmation of correct target location as a possible reason to decrease the overall time of the surgical intervention and to reduce the risk of possible complications related to brain tissue trauma.

Corresponding to this surgical concept we found a sustained improvement in PD-associated motor disability (UPDRS), a reduction of postoperative L-Dopa respectively L-Dopa-equivalent medication and a minimizing of levodopa-induced motor complications, which is confirmed by other study results. Despite of other surgical concepts of target definition, which published elsewhere, the MR-based STN localization leads to comparable results in both groups.

The STN is a biconvex lens-shaped structure, which can be visualized as a hypointense region by T2w MRI. Described by Yelnik and Percheron, 1979, STN as a relatively small region of approximately 735 mm³ is obliquely oriented along the three anatomical axis of the space, which means approximately 20° oblique to the horizontal plane, 35° to the sagittal plane, and approximately 55° to the frontal plane (Yelnik & Percheron, 1979). As a consequence the STN has three anatomical characteristics, which make its localization difficult: it is lens shaped, relatively small, and oblique. For these reasons, the position of STN cannot be simply determined by viewing a single planar plane, but rather requires a precise and reproducible 3D reconstruction of its entire extent and a clear differentiation from the surrounding tissue. Besides the anatomical peculiarities the STN shows interindividual variations in size, shape and dimension, which complicated the positioning of electrodes basing on statistical and anatomical coordinates. In this study we used different MR modalities (T1w, T2w, 1.5mT vs. 3mT) to define the target point. Following postprocessing allowing a detailed visualization in all three sections of the space and perpendicularly along the planned trajectories, using excellent contrast between hypointense structure of STN and Nc. ruber and the hyperintense tissue in the surrounding. With the use of 3mT MRI a high resolution of basal cerebral structures, including the target area of STN and its neighbouring structures, could be achieved. Criteria for the following placement of microelectrodes were the longest medial-lateral and ventral-posterior diameter of STN and the ventral border of the red nucleus. The central trajectory was aimed and located immediately lateral to the anterior aspect of the Nc. ruber in the axial plane with regard to the patient's anatomy. MER and macrostimulation were used for electrophysiological respectively clinical validation of chosen trajectories for final electrodes. MER obtained by electrophysiological examination were consistent with other reports of bursting and non-bursting activities (Hutchison et al., 1998; Raeva & Lukashev, 1993) and correlated in the majority of tested trajectories with the typical STN signature in frequency and amplitude. Microrecording results were limited by the typical activity patterns of neighbouring structures of the zona inserta, substantia nigra and the background activity of the basal cerebral structures as well.

The image guided placement of micro- and final electrodes implicates the preoperative fixation of the stereotaxic frame just before image acquisition hours before surgery. Unfortunately most of these classic stereotaxic frames (weight: 2000 to 2500 g) are really heavy and uncomfortable during it's fixation on the patients skull. During image acquisition, planning and surgical procedure all patients are free of L-Dopa medication to guarantee a reliable neurological testing during electrode positioning and following clinical testing. Stress, medication free interval and tremor-associated disability enforce possible motion artefacts in the acquisition of planning image data sets. This movement theoretically reduces the accuracy of image coregistration between image modalities.

Following preoperative postprocessing procedure including image fusion and definition of electrode trajectories is time consuming - to be just in time on the day of surgery is stressfull for patients and surgeons and can be a logistic problem, which is difficult to measure.

Beside the fixation of the patient´s head on the table via special head holders conventional functional neurosurgery requires the adjustment of all axis of the space corresponding to the target and entry coordinates using the microdrive and a special target arcl. A re-checking is following using by the target arch simulator, which gives additional safety, but which is time consuming. After finishing the dominant side all the equipment has to be removed, readjusted and readapted for the second side, which delay the surgery additionally and which implicates moments of inaccuracies. In the consequence, the accuracy of "static" image guided devices decreases with the time of surgery secondary to the intraoperative brain shift as a result of a) loss of cerebrospinal fluid (CSF), b) gravity, c) anaesthesiological procedure and d) brain-immanent characteristics. Confirmed by own experiences a tissue shift even in the region of STN could be documented exemplarily in the end of a hours lasting routine DBS procedure by vectorshift deformation analysis, which expressly underline the requirement of a stringent surgery. As a result of diverse shift studies it´s accepted, that long lasting procedures can dipose progressive CSF loss via burr hole trepanation and brain shift associated inaccuracies even in the middle of the brain. In the consequence, all factors, disposing shift associated inaccuracies should be prevented strictly. Microrecording and macrostimulation are relatively standardised steps and can help to compensate the mentioned inaccuracies electrophysiologically. Both neurosurgical steps are the preconditions for the following positioning of the final electrode.

In this series the mean number of active electrodes was with 6.7 (group I) and 7.1 (group II) per patient should be very good, but is confirmed by other studies. In our opinion the slight difference of the mean number of active electrodes between both groups is a possibly result of a better resolution of anatomical structures and improved signal-to-noise ratio by 3 T MRI, especially in the target region and can be the reason for a shorter surgical time. In our study intraoperative MER was an essential tool to find an optimal target point for the macrostimulation, which can reduce the surgeon's uncertainty and increases the procedure's safety. Macrostimulation was performed only in this macroelectrode, in which the cellular activity characteristics of the STN have been identified. The criteria for changing stimulation electrode were the missing motor effect of macrostimulation and persistent stimulation-induced side effects, including paresis, sensible sensations or dyskinesia. Correct anatomical and functional target – namely where the best clinical result with a partial or complete relief of symptoms – were the base for the actual placement of the permanent electrode.

As a consequence of preoperative postprocessing and following planning procedure the functional coordinates were comparable in both groups and differed only slightly, especially the x-coordinates, which were ± 11.25 in group I and ± 10.4 in group II. This correlates possibly with a changed selection of the best track for the permanent electrode placement from the central position (48%) in group I to the anterior (41.7%) and central (37.5%) position in group II. Maybe this is an indication for the phenomenon that a smaller distance from the target point to the AC-PC line correlates with a good clinical response stimulating the anterior part of the Nc. subthalamicus. However, both study groups are too small to conclude a strict and reliable tendency.

Corresponding to this surgical concept we found a sustained improvement in PD-associated motor disability (UPDRS, part III), which is confirmed by Pollo et al., 2007, and Kleiner-Fisman et al., 2006, presenting meta-analysis of outcomes from 1993 until 2004.

The medication doses could be reduced to the same extent in both groups and were in the range reported in the literature (Beric et al., 2001; Limousin et al., 1998; Minguez-Castellanos et al., 2005; Okun et al., 2005; Russmann et al., 2004). Differences in preoperative image acquisition (1.5 T, 3 T), postprocessing and defined target coordinates and chosen electrode tracks were not associated with a definite improvement of motor response and drug reduction, which would justify the use of 3 T MRI absolutely.

4. Conclusions

Acquisition of T2w 3 T MRI for following planning procedure is a useful tool to visualize the target region and anatomical landmarks with a high fidelity of detailed information. Microrecording is an excellent and reliable method to validate the target area intraoperatively by registration of typical STN signatures. Over and above that, it allows an identification of the longest segment of STN, which we preferred as the electrode position for macrostimulation and for placement of permanent STN-electrode. With the use of 3 T MRI data for image postprocessing and planning procedure the visualization of the target point – the STN – could be improved and allowed a high precision in the definition of target and entry coordinates of the virtual trajectory. Macrostimulation via macroeletrodes confirmed the target point and was used to detect any side effects for further stimulation. The macrostimulation and intraoperative testing guaranteed a proper placement of both electrodes, expecting a high rate of successful surgeries and permanent functional effects.

With our study we could confirm an encouraging response of PD-associated movement disorders. Besides the neuroradiological, physiological and neurosurgical techniques and procedures, the most important prerequisite is the optimal visualization of the target area, which can be achieved by high-resolution MRI. In the consequence using 3 T MRI series is one way to increase the surgeons and patients safety and to support an optimal electrode placement.

But, this study is not suitable to conclude, that a better visualization of the STN is also associated with a further clinical improvement of motor response and reduction of L-dopa, which is known in conventional functional neurosurgery using 1.5 T MRI. Further studies should be initiated to find a better conclusion. Up to this point, the choice of method should depend on the technical resources, preferences and experiences of each centre.

5. References

Agid Y: Continuous high frequency stimulation of deep brain structures in brain pathology. Brain Res Bull 1999, 50:475

Anderson VC, Burchiel KJ, Hogarth P, Favre J, Hammerstad JP: Pallidal vs subthalamic nucleus deep brain stimulation in Parkinson disease. Arch Neurol 2005, 62:554-560

Benabid AL, Benazzouz A, Hoffmann D, Limousin P, Krack P, Pollak P: Long-term electrical inhibition of deep brain targets in movement disorders. Mov Disord 1998, 13:119-125

Benazzouz A, Hallett M: Mechanism of action of deep brain stimulation. Neurology 2000, 55:13-16

Beric A, Kelly PJ, Rezai A et al.. Complications of Deep Brain Stimulation Surgery. Stereotact Funct Neurosurg2001;77:73-78

Targeting the Subthalamic Nucleus for Deep Brain Stimulation in Parkinson Disease: The Impact of High Field
Strength MRI

83

DeLong MR, Wichmann T: Deep brain stimulation for Parkinson's disease. Ann Neurol 2001, 49:142-143

Dowsey-Limousin P, Fraix V, Benabid AL, Pollak P: Deep brain stimulation in Parkinson's disease. Funct Neurol 2001, 16:67-71

Dujardin K, Defebvre L, Krystkowiak P, Blond S, Destèe A. Influence of chronic bilateral stimulation of the subthalamic nucleus on cognitive function in Parkinson's disease. J Neurol. 2001; 248,603-611

Hariz MI, Bergenheim AT (1993) Clinical evaluation of computed tomography-guided versus ventriculography-guided thalamotomy for movement disorders. Acta Neurochir 58 : 53-55

Hariz MI, Fodstad H: Deep brain stimulation in Parkinsons's disease. N Engl J Med 2002, 346:452-453

Hariz, MI, Bergenheim, AT (1990) A comparative study on ventriculographic and computerized tomography-guided determinations of brain targets in functional stereotaxis. J Neurosurg 73 : 565-571

Hutchison WD, Allan RJ, Opitz, H et al: Neurophysiological identification of the subthalamic nucleus in surgery for Parkinson's disease. Ann Neurol 44:622-628, 1998

Kleiner-Fisman G, Herzog J, Fisman DN, Tamma F, Lyons KE, Rahwa R, Lang AE, Deuschl G: Subthalamic nucleus deep brain stimulation: summary and meta-analysis of outcomes. Mov Disord 2006, 21:290-304

Koller WC, Lyons KE, Wilkinson SB, Troster AI, Pahwa R: Longterm safety and efficacy of unilateral deep brain stimulation of the thalamus in essential tremor. Mov Disord 2001, 16:464-468

Kopper F, Volkmann J, Müller D, Mehdorn M, Deuschl G. High-frequency deep brain stimulation in the treatment for Parkinson's disease, tremor and dystonia. Der Nervenarzt. 2003;74:709-725

Krack P, Pollak P, Limousin P et al.. Subthalamic nucleus or internal pallidal stimulation in young onset Parkinson's disease Brain. 1998; 121, 451 – 457

Krause M, Fogel W, Heck A, Hacke W, Bonsanto M, Trenkwalder C, Tronnier V: Deep brain stimulation for the treatment of Parkinson's disease: subthalamic nucleus versus globus pallidum internus. J Neurol Neurosurg Psychiatry 2001, 70:464-470

Kupsch A, Earl C (1999) Neurosurgical intervention in the treatment of ideopathic Parkinson disease: neurostimulation and neural implantation. J Mol Med 77 : 178-84

Limousin P, Krack P, Pollack P et al.. Electrical stimulation of the subthalamic nucleus in advanced Parkinson's disease. N Engl J Med. 1998;339:1105-1111

Lopiano L, Rizzone M, Bergamasco B et al.. Deep brain stimulation of the subthalamic nucleus in PD: an analysis of the exclusion causes. Journal of the Neurological Sciences. 2002;195;167-170

Lopiano L, Rizzone M, Bergamasco B, Tavella A, Torre E, Perozzo P, Valentini MC, Lanotte M: Deep brain stimulation of the subthalamic nucleus: clinical effectiveness and safety. Neurology 2001, 56:552-554

Martinez-Martin P, Valldeoriola F, Tolosa E et al.. Bilateral Subthalamic Nucleus Stimulation and Quality of Life in Advanced Parkinson's Disease. Movement Disorders. 2002;17, 372 – 377

Minguez-Castellanos A, Escamilla-Sevilla F, Katati MJ, Martin-Linares JM, Meersmans M, Ortega-Moreno A, Arjona V: Different patterns of medication ch'ange after subthalamic or pallidal stimulation for Parkinson's disease: target related effect or selection bias? J Neurol Neurosurg Psychiatry 2005, 76:34-39

Okun MS, Tagliati M, Pourfar M, Fernandes HH, Rodriguez RL, Alterman RL, Foote KD: Management of referred deep brain stimulation failures: a retrospective analysis from 2 movement disorders centers. Arch Neurol 2005, 62:1250-1255

Pollo C, Vingerhoets F, Pralong E, Ghika J, Maeder P, Meuli R, Thiran JP, Villemure JG: Localization of electrodes in the subthalamic nucleus on magnetic resonance imaging. J Neurosurg 2007, 106:36-44

Raeva S, Lukashev A, Lashin A: Unit activity in human thalamic reticularis neuron. I. Spontaneous activity. Electroencephalogr Clin Neurophysiol 79:133-140, 1991

Raeva S, Lukashev A: Unit activity in human thalamic reticularis neuron. II. Activity evoked by significant and non-significant verbal or sensory stimuli. Electroencephalogr Clin Neurophysiol 86:110-122, 1993

Russmann H, Ghiera J, Combrement P, Villemure JG, Bogousslavsky J, Burkhard PR, Vingerhoets FJ: L-dopa-induced dyskinesia improvement after STN-DBS depends upon medication reduction. Neurology 2004, 63:153-155

Vesper J, Klostermann F, Stockhammer F, Funk T, Brock M: Results of chronic subthalamic nucleus (STN) stimulation for Parkinson's disease – a one-year follow-up study. Surg Neurol 2002, 57:306-313

Volkmann J, Allert N, Voges J, Weiss PH, Freund HJ, Sturm V: Safety and efficacy of pallidal or subthalamic nucleus stimulation in advanced PD. Neurology 2001, 56:548-551

Yelnik J, Percheron G: Subthalamic neurons in primates: a quantitative and comparative analysis. Neuroscience 4:1717-1743, 1979

5

Cognitive and Behavioural Changes After Deep Brain Stimulation of the Subthalamic Nucleus in Parkinson's Disease

Antonio Daniele, Pietro Spinelli and Chiara Piccininni
Istituto di Neurologia,
Università Cattolica, Rome,
Italy

1. Introduction

In patients with Parkinson's disease, cognitive impairment is common, may be detectable in early disease stages, even in young patients, and may progress to overt dementia. In addition, a variety of psychiatric and behavioural symptoms may occur in Parkinsonian patients, including depression, apathy, anxiety, visual hallucinations, sleep disorders, impulse control disorders, punding and the dopamine dysregulation syndrome. The cognitive and behavioural symptoms observed in these patients may be part of the non-motor symptoms of Parkinson's disease, which can appear in various phases of the disease course.

Various mechanisms might be involved in the pathogenesis of cognitive and behavioral symptoms in Parkinson's disease. Cognitive and behavioural symptoms observed in Parkinsonian patients might be related to disruption of various circuits involving dopaminergic, noradrenergic, cholinergic, and serotonergic systems (Candy et al., 1983; Mayeux et al., 1984; Cash et al., 1987; Mattay et al., 2002). Moreover, in patients with Parkinson's disease and dementia, neuropathological examination (Xuereb et al., 1990; Hughes et al., 1993) may show in several cortical areas the presence of Lewy Bodies (the histopathological hallmark of Parkinson's disease) or neurodegenerative lesions typical of Alzheimer's disease (amyloid plaques and neurofibrillary tangles). Furthermore, in patients with Parkinson's disease pharmacological treatment with anti-Parkinsonian dopaminergic drugs may have beneficial or detrimental effects on distinct cognitive functions (Malapani et al., 1994; Kulisevsky et al., 1996; Mattay et al., 2002) and may also play a role in the development of some behavioural disorders.

Among the cognitive deficits which may be detected in patients with Parkinson's disease, deficits of executive functions (planning, problem solving, set-shifting), mediated by disruption of neural circuits involving the frontal lobes and the basal ganglia, are the most common in both early disease phases and in patients with advanced Parkinson's disease (Morris et al., 1988; Cooper et al., 1991; Robbins et al., 1994; Taylor et al., 1986; Cools et al., 2001; Green et al., 2002).

In addition, memory deficits (Taylor et al., 1986; Harrington et al., 1990; Cooper et al., 1991; Robbins et al., 1994; Dubois and Pillon, 1997), deficits of visuo-spatial cognitive functions

(Boller et al., 1984; Hovestadt et al., 1987; Ransmayr et al., 1987), impairment on language tasks of verbal fluency (Matison et al., 1982; Cooper et al., 1991) and tasks of oral naming (Peran et al., 2003) may occur in individual Parkinsonian patients since early phases and become more frequent in advanced Parkinson's disease (Green et al., 2002).

As to memory deficits, different studies reported in Parkinsonian patients an impairment of episodic memory (Taylor et al., 1986), verbal short-term memory (Cooper et al., 1991), spatial short-term memory (Robbins et al., 1994), and procedural memory (Harrington et al., 1990). In patients with Parkinson's disease and dementia, the pattern of neuropsychological impairment may differ in distinct patient subgroups.

A subgroup of Parkinsonian patients, in which neurodegenerative lesions in the cerebral cortex seem to be less remarkable (Xuereb et al., 1990), may show a pattern of subcortical dementia, mainly characterized by remarkable deficits of executive functions (Litvan et al., 1991), associated with mild to moderate deficits of episodic long-term memory (Helkala et al., 1988) and, in some patients, deficits of visuo-spatial cognitive functions (Mohr et al., 1995), with relative sparing of linguistic and praxic functions (Dubois and Pillon, 1997). In another subgroup of patients with Parkinson's disease and dementia, in which neurodegenerative lesions in the cerebral cortex are more remarkable, in addition to the previously described neuropsychological pattern of subcortical dementia, it is possible to observe a an impairment of other cognitive functions mediated by various cortical areas, namely an impairment of linguistic and praxic functions and severe deficits of episodic long-term memory (Mohr et al., 1990; Mohr et al., 1995; Marsh, 2000).

As to psychiatric and behavioural symptoms which may be observed in patients with Parkinson's disease, depression, apathy, anxiety and visual hallucinations are the most common manifestations. Depressive syndromes (major depression and dysthymic disorder) may occur in up to 45% of Parkinsonian patients (Burn, 2002). Both psychosocial and neurobiological factors might be involved in the pathogenesis of depressive syndromes in Parkinson's disease. The role of psychosocial factors (such as a psychological reaction to motor disability) is suggested by studies reporting a significant correlation between severity of depressive symptoms and severity of motor symptoms (Gotham et al., 1986), while other investigations support the role of neurobiological factors such as a disruption of dopaminergic (Torack e Morris, 1988; Mayberg e Solomon, 1995), noradrenergic (Cubo et al., 2000; Menza et al., 2009) and serotonergic (Paulus e Jellinger, 1991) systems, which may occur in early phases of Parkinson's disease (Braak et al., 2004) and might result in the appearance of depressive symptoms. In some Parkinsonian patients, depressive symptoms may occur some years before the appearance of Parkinsonian motor symptoms, in agreement with the hypothesis of a critical role of neurobiological factors (Aarsland et al., 2009).

Apathy, which is characterised by a reduction in interest, motivation and initiative in daily living activities, is common in patients with Parkinson's disease and was detected in 17% to 70% of Parkinsonian patients in different studies (Leentjens et al., 2008; Pedersen et al., 2009). Although the pathogenic mechanisms involved in apathy in Parkinson's disease need to be further clarified, a dysfunction of the "limbic" circuit (Alexander et al., 1986) of the basal ganglia (which involve the ventral striatum, the anterior part of the cingulate gyrus and the mesial orbitofrontal cortex) might play a critical role.

Psychotic symptoms such as delusions and hallucinations are common in patients with Parkinson's disease and may occur in up to 26% of patients (Sanchez-Ramoz et al., 1996). In patients with Parkinson's disease, hallucinations and delusions may result from multiple pathogenic factors. Although these psychotic symptoms may be induced by the administration of dopaminergic anti-Parkinsonian drugs (Factor et al., 1995; Valldeoriola et al., 1997), they may occur also in Parkinsonian patients who do not receive any pharmacological treatment (Factor et al., 1995). The prevalence of hallucinations and delusions does increase with disease progression. Moreover, cognitive impairment is usually more marked in Parkinsonian patients with hallucinations as compared with Parkinsonian patients without hallucinations (Katzen et al., 2010). Visual hallucinations are the most frequent, are characterised by visions of people or animals, and are usually perceived as unpleasant.

Anxiety is also common in patients with Parkinson's disease, although epidemiological studies focussed on the prevalence of anxiety in these patients are still needed. In a recent study carried out in patients with Parkinson's disease in early stages, the prevalence of anxiety was about 27% (Bugalho et al., 2012).

Impulse control disorders (Ambermoon et al., 2011), punding and the dopamine dysregulation syndrome (Lim et al., 2009) have been increasingly recognized in recent years in patients with Parkinson's disease.

It has been reported that up to 13.6% of Parkinsonian patients (Weintraub et al, 2010) may develop behavioural changes due to a reduced impulse control (pathological gambling, hypersexuality, compulsive eating and buying/shopping). Such impulse control disorders may have dramatic implications for the personal life of the patient and for the patient's family.

In Parkinsonian patients, dopamine replacement therapy might play a role in the pathophysiology of impulse control disorders, by inducing an overstimulation of the mesolimbic dopaminergic system, which is critically involved in response to reward and motivation (Demetriades et al, 2011).

It has been suggested that in patients with Parkinson's disease the risk to develop impulse control disorders (Demetriades et al, 2011) may be increased by several demographic and clinical variables (younger age of onset of Parkinson's disease, treatment with dopamine agonists, male gender, pre-existing psychiatric disorders).

In Parkinsonian patients, the dopamine dysregulation syndrome is characterized by an overuse of dopaminergic anti-Parkinsonian drugs, resulting in the compulsive assumption of higher daily doses than those required to treat motor symptoms (Giovannoni et al., 2000).

Punding is a behavioural disorder in which the patient is frequently engaged in repetitive, stereotyped, non-goal-oriented activities. In patients with Parkinson's disease, punding may be triggered by dopaminergic anti-Parkinsonian drugs.

Deep brain stimulation of the subthalamic nucleus is an established neurosurgical procedure in the treatment of Parkinson's disease, which may remarkably improve the motor symptoms and quality of life in Parkinsonian patients (Hamani et al., 2005).

Deep brain stimulation of the subthalamic nucleus is more effective than best medical therapy in improving Parkinsonian motor symptoms and dyskinesias (Hamani et al., 2005) and allows to obtain a long-lasting decrease of the daily doses of anti-Parkinsonian medications. However, a worsening of axial motor symptoms (postural instability, freezing of gait, difficulties in articulation of speech) may be frequently observed at long-term follow-up, as reported in a 8-year follow-up study carried out in 20 Parkinsonian patients who underwent bilateral deep brain stimulation of the subthalamic nucleus (Fasano et al., 2010).

While the beneficial effects of bilateral deep brain stimulation of the subthalamic nucleus on motor symptoms in patients with advanced PD have been clearly analyzed by several studies, the effects of deep brain stimulation of the subthalamic nucleus on cognition and behaviour may at least partially differ among different studies and need to be further investigated.

2. Cognitive performance in Parkinsonian patients treated by deep brain stimulation of the subthalamic nucleus

Several investigations have assessed cognitive functioning in patients with Parkinson's disease treated by deep brain stimulation of the subthalamic nucleus, with variable duration of postoperative follow-up in different studies. In these investigations, statistical comparisons were made between preoperative (baseline) performance of Parkinsonian patients on neuropsychological tasks and postoperative performance on the same tasks.

Across all neuropsychological studies assessing cognitive functioning in patients with Parkinson's disease treated by deep brain stimulation of the subthalamic nucleus, a consistently reported finding is a postoperative decline on tasks of phonological and semantic verbal fluency (Ardouin et al. 1999; Pillon et al. 2000, Daniele et al. 2003; Funkiewiez et al. 2004; Parsons et al., 2006), which was detected already few months after surgery in some studies and gradually increased over time in studies with long-term follow-up (Contarino et al., 2007; Fasano et al., 2010).

On the other hand, different studies reported less consistent findings on other cognitive tasks, including tasks of episodic memory and working memory and tasks assessing frontal cognitive functions (Parson et al., 2006).

2.1 Performance of Parkinsonian patients treated by deep brain stimulation of the subthalamic nucleus on tasks of verbal fluency

In patients affected by Parkinson's disease who underwent deep brain stimulation of the subthalamic nucleus, a postoperative decline on tasks of phonological and semantic verbal fluency has been consistently reported by all neuropsychological investigations. Such decline on performance on verbal fluency tasks has been usually detected few months after the surgical intervention and has been observed in patients with 1-year (Pillon et al., 2000; Daniele et al., 2003), 3-year (Funkiewiz et al., 2004), 5-year (Contarino et al., 2007; Fasano et al., 2010), and 8-year follow-up (Fasano et al., 2010). A recent study aimed at assessing long-term motor and cognitive outcome 8 years after implants for deep brain stimulation of the subthalamic nucleus in 20 patients with Parkinson's disease (Fasano et al., 2010) detected a decline on phonological verbal fluency task, which was slightly more pronounced 8 years than 5 years after surgery.

In this study, 8 years after surgery performance on a phonological verbal fluency task could be assessed in 16 Parkinsonian patients. Interestingly, the analysis of raw scores (adjusted for age and educational level) obtained by individual Parkinsonian patients on the letter verbal fluency task at 8-year follow-up showed that only 2 out of 16 patients (12.5%) performed below the normal range and 1 patient (6.2%) scored around the cut-off score, while 13 out 16 patients (81.2%) performed in the normal range (Fasano et al., 2010). These latter findings suggest that in selected cohorts of Parkinsonian patients treated by deep brain stimulation of the subthalamic nucleus the statistically significant decline on verbal fluency tasks observed as a group effect is associated with large interindividual variability (Contarino et al., 2007) and in some individual Parkinsonian patients might be not remarkable.

It should be pointed out that a poor performance on tasks of verbal fluency is frequently observed also in patients with Parkinson's disease patients treated by pallidotomy, especially after left-sided pallidotomy (Troster et al., 2003) and even in patients with Parkinson's disease who are not treated by neurosurgical procedures (Matison et al., 1982).

Recently, some investigations have attempted to compare performance on verbal fluency tasks in two different groups of patients with Parkinson's disease, namely patients treated by deep brain stimulation of the subthalamic nucleus versus Parkinsonian patients treated only by anti-Parkinsonian drugs (Zangaglia et al., 2009; Castelli et al., 2010; Williams et al., 2011). Such comparative studies consistently found that performance on verbal fluency tasks was significantly better in Parkinsonian patients treated only by anti-Parkinsonian drugs, as compared to patients who underwent deep brain stimulation of the subthalamic nucleus and were followed-up for 6 months (Witt et al., 2008), 1 year (Castelli et al., 2010), 2 years (Williams et al. 2011) and 3 years (Zangaglia et al., 2009).

In a randomized multicentre study (Witt et al., 2008), 123 patients with advanced Parkinson's disease and motor fluctuations were randomly assigned to have deep brain stimulation of the subthalamic nucleus or the best medical treatment for Parkinson's disease (according to the German Society of Neurology guidelines) and underwent neuropsychological and psychiatric examinations to detect possible changes 6 months after surgery, as compared to baseline. Sixty patients were randomly assigned to receive deep brain stimulation of the subthalamic nucleus and 63 patients to have best medical treatment.

After 6 months, the group of Parkinsonian patients treated by deep brain stimulation of the subthalamic nucleus showed a significantly greater decline on tasks of phonological and semantic verbal fluency, as compared to the group of patients treated with the best medical treatment. These findings suggest that the impairment on verbal fluency tasks observed in patients who underwent subthalamic implants is not simply due to disease progression, but might be rather due to the neurosurgical intervention.

In a prospective 3-year follow-up study (Zangaglia et al., 2009), 32 Parkinsonian patients underwent deep brain stimulation of the subthalamic nucleus, while 33 Parkinsonian patients, even though eligible for this surgical procedure, declined surgery and were treated only by anti-Parkinsonian drugs. In this latter study, as compared to the group of patients treated with the best medical treatment, the group of Parkinsonian patients treated by deep brain stimulation of the subthalamic nucleus showed at 1-month and 3-year follow-up a significantly greater decline on a task of phonological verbal fluency.

In conclusion, the postoperative decline on verbal fluency tasks in patients with Parkinson's disease treated by deep brain stimulation of the subthalamic nucleus does not seem to have clinically meaningful effects on daily living activities, even in patients with long-term follow-up (Contarino et al., 2007).

Various hypotheses have been proposed to account for the postoperative decline on tasks of verbal fluency observed in patients with Parkinson's disease treated by deep brain stimulation of the subthalamic nucleus. On one hand, it has been suggested that the postoperative decline on such fluency tasks might be due to the neurosurgical procedure, namely to surgical microlesions affecting cortical-basal ganglionic circuits involved in word retrieval processes (Troster et al., 2003). This hypothesis is supported by the observation that the decline on verbal fluency tasks in Parkinsonian patients has been usually detected in very early phases after the subthalamic implant. An alternative hypothesis suggests that is the stimulation of the subthalamic nucleus which might lead to a decreased activity of various cortical areas in the left cerebral hemisphere (inferior frontal, insular and temporal areas), giving rise to a decreased performance on verbal fluency tasks (Schroeder et al. 2003).

2.2 Performance of Parkinsonian patients treated by deep brain stimulation of the subthalamic nucleus on tasks of episodic memory and abstract reasoning

As suggested by a meta-analysis on neuropsychological studies in patients with Parkinson's disease treated by deep brain stimulation of the subthalamic nucleus (Parsons et al., 2006), a statistically significant but small decline of postoperative performance on tasks of episodic verbal memory has been reported in some investigations (Alegret et al., 2001; Daniele et al., 2003; Dujardin et al., 2001; Jahanshahi et al., 2000; Pillon et al., 2000; Saint-Cyr et al., 2000; Trepanier et al., 2000), but not in others. Such postoperative decline on episodic verbal memory tasks was detectable already 3 months after surgery in some studies (Alegret et al., 2001; Daniele et al., 2003), while in one cohort became not statistically significant at 1-year follow-up (Daniele et al., 2003).

In a recent study which attempted to compare performance on various neuropsychological tasks in two different groups of patients with Parkinson's disease followed-up for 12 months, namely 105 patients treated by deep brain stimulation of the subthalamic nucleus versus 40 Parkinsonian patients treated only by anti-Parkinsonian drugs (Smedding et al., 2011), performance at 6 and 12 months of postoperative follow-up on tasks of episodic verbal memory (immediate and delayed recall of the Rey's Auditory Verbal Learning Test) was significantly poorer in Parkinsonian patients who underwent subthalamic implants, as compared to patients treated only by anti-Parkinsonian drugs.

As to studies with long-term follow-up, a statistically significant but slight decline on episodic verbal memory tasks (immediate and delayed recall of the Rey's Auditory Verbal Learning Test) as compared to preoperative baseline was detected 8 years after subthalamic implants (Fasano et al., 2010).

However, in the cohort of 16 Parkinsonian patients followed up in such long-term study (Fasano et al., 2010), the analysis of individual raw scores (adjusted for age and educational level) showed that at 8-year follow-up on the immediate recall subtest of the Rey's Auditory Verbal Learning Test only 3 out of 16 Parkinsonian patients (18.7%) performed below the normal range and 1 out of 16 patients (6.2%) scored around the cut-off score discriminating between normal and pathological performance, while 12 out of 16 patients (75%) performed in the normal range.

In the same cohort, on the delayed recall subtest of the Rey's Auditory Verbal Learning Test, only 3 out of 16 Parkinsonian patients (18.7%) at 8-year follow-up performed below the normal range, while 13 out of 16 Parkinsonian patients (81.2%) performed in the normal range (Fasano et al., 2010).

These latter individual data suggest that in selected cohorts of Parkinsonian patients treated by deep brain stimulation of the subthalamic nucleus the statistically significant decline on episodic verbal memory tasks observed as a group effect is associated with a large interindividual variability and might be not remarkable in some individual Parkinsonian patients.

A statistically significant but slight decline on a task of abstract reasoning (Raven's Progressive Matrices '47) was reported in neuropsychological studies in the same cohort of Parkinsonian patients treated by deep brain stimulation of the subthalamic nucleus, which were assessed 5 years (Contarino et al., 2007) and 8 years after surgery (Fasano et al., 2010).

However, at 5-year follow-up the analysis of individual raw scores (adjusted for age and educational level) obtained by 11 individual Parkinsonian patients showed that on such task of abstract reasoning (Raven's Progressive Matrices '47) only 2 out of 11 Parkinsonian patients performed slightly below the normal range, while the remaining 9 patients performed in the normal range (Contarino et al., 2007).

Similarly, at 8-year follow-up the analysis of the raw scores (adjusted for age and educational level) obtained by 16 individual Parkinsonian patients on Raven's Progressive Matrices '47 showed that only 1 out of 16 patients scored around the cut-off score, while the remaining 15 patients performed in the normal range (Fasano et al., 2010).

These individual data suggest that in selected cohorts of Parkinsonian patients treated by deep brain stimulation of the subthalamic nucleus the statistically significant decline on tasks of abstract reasoning observed as a group effect at long-term follow-up might be not remarkable in individual Parkinsonian patients.

2.3 Performance of Parkinsonian patients treated by deep brain stimulation of the subthalamic nucleus on tasks assessing cognitive functions mediated by the frontal lobes

In patients with Parkinson's disease treated by deep brain stimulation of the subthalamic nucleus, different effects have been described on neuropsychological tasks assessing distinct cognitive functions mediated by the frontal lobes.

On one hand, various studies reported after subthalamic implants an impaired performance on frontal tasks assessing response inhibition, such as the interference subtest of the Stroop test (Jahanshahi et al., 2000; Schroeder et al., 2002; Witt et al., 2004), in ON-stimulation condition as compared to the OFF-stimulation condition.

A positron emission tomography study showed that such impaired performance on the interference subtest of the Stroop test in the on-stimulation condition was associated with decreased activation in both the right anterior cingulate cortex and the right ventral striatum (Schroeder et al., 2002).

In a previously mentioned randomized multicentre study (Witt et al. , 2008) carried out in 123 Parkinsonian patients who were randomly assigned to receive deep brain stimulation of the subthalamic nucleus (n =60) or to have best medical treatment (n=63), as compared to the best medical treatment group the group of patients treated by deep brain stimulation showed 6 months after surgery a significantly greater decline on several variables of the Stroop test. This finding might be accounted for by a dysfunction of neural circuits involving the basal ganglia and the frontal lobes, which might play a critical role in response selection (Witt et al., 2008) and response inhibition.

On the other hand, in patients with Parkinson's disease treated by deep brain stimulation of the subthalamic nucleus an improved postoperative performance has been reported in early phases of follow-up (6 six months after surgery) up to 26 months on neuropsychological frontal tasks assessing cognitive flexibility, such as the Modified Wisconsin Card Sorting Test (Jahanshahi et al., 2000; Daniele et al., 2003) and tasks of random number generation (Witt et al., 2004).

In a neuropsychological study carried out in 20 Parkinsonian patients who underwent bilateral deep brain stimulation of the subthalamic nucleus (Daniele et al., 2003), patients were tested 3 months after surgery with stimulators switched off, while 6 and 12 months after surgery they were tested with stimulators switched on. In this study, an improved performance on a task of cognitive flexibility (Modified Wisconsin Card Sorting Test) was detected 6 and 12 months after surgery, when stimulators were switched on. It was hypothesised that such improved performance on the Modified Wisconsin Card Sorting Test could arise either from a genuine improvement of a specific frontal executive function such as cognitive flexibility (i.e. set-shifting ability) due to subthalamic implants or, alternatively, from a practice effect resulting from the repeated administration of the same cognitive task over time (Daniele et al., 2003).

In a study carried out in 23 Parkinsonian patients who underwent bilateral deep brain stimulation of the subthalamic nucleus and were tested 6 to 12 months after surgery with stimulators switched on or off in random order (Witt et al., 2004), in the ON-stimulation condition there was a poorer performance on a task of response inhibition (interference subtest of the Stroop test) and an improved performance on a task of cognitive flexibility (random number generation), as compared to the OFF-stimulation condition.

These findings are at least partially consistent with the results of a preliminary study carried out in 7 Parkinsonian patients treated by bilateral deep brain stimulation of the subthalamic nucleus (Jahanshahi et al., 2000), who were tested at variable intervals after surgery (4 to 26 months after surgery, with a mean of 11.7 months) with stimulators switched ON or OFF in random order. In this latter study, in the ON-stimulation condition there was a better performance on tasks of cognitive flexibility (random number generation, Modified Wisconsin Card Sorting Test), as compared to the OFF-stimulation condition.

On the whole, these studies suggest that stimulation of the subthalamic nucleus might have different effects on distinct neural circuits involving the basal ganglia and the frontal lobes, resulting in a potential improvement of performance on neuropsychological tasks assessing cognitive flexibility (set-shifting ability) and a potential impairment of performance on neuropsychological tasks assessing response inhibition.

As to studies with long-term follow-up, a statistically significant but slight decline on a task of cognitive flexibility (number of correct criteria discovered on the Modified Wisconsin Card Sorting Test) was detected 8 years after subthalamic implants, as compared to preoperative baseline (Fasano et al., 2010). In this study, as to the number of correct criteria on the Modified Wisconsin Card Sorting Test, the analysis of individual raw scores of a cohort of 15 Parkinsonian patients showed that at 8-year postoperative follow-up 6 out of 15 patients (40%) performed below the normal range, while the remaining 9 patients (60%) performed in the normal range (Fasano et al., 2010).

Eight years after surgery, Parkinsonian patients with a worsening of postoperative performance (increased number of total errors as compared to baseline) on the Modified Wisconsin Card Sorting Test showed significantly higher scores on items assessing postural stability (namely, a poorer postural stability), as compared to patients in which postoperative performance on the Modified Wisconsin Card Sorting Test (number of total errors as compared to baseline) was improved or unchanged (Fasano et al., 2010).

As to decision-making processes, in which the subthalamic nucleus and prefrontal cortical areas might play a critical role, some studies reported after deep brain stimulation of the subthalamic nucleus (Frank et al., 2007) a reduced ability of Parkinsonian patients to slow down their decisions in high-conflict conditions (namely, an increased impulsivity), while other studies detected an improved performance on tasks of reward-based decision learning (VanWouve et al, 2011).

2.4 Long-term cognitive follow-up in patients treated by deep brain stimulation of the subthalamic nucleus

To summarise the results of the previously mentioned study which assessed motor and cognitive outcome in Parkinsonian patients 8 years after subthalamic implants (Fasano et al., 2010), this investigation reported a statistically significant decline on a phonological verbal fluency task and a statistically significant but slight decline on tasks of abstract reasoning (Raven's Progressive Matrices '47), episodic verbal memory (immediate and delayed recall of the Rey's Auditory Verbal Learning Test), executive functioning (number of correct criteria on the Modified Wisconsin Card Sorting Test).

2.5 Prevalence of dementia in patients treated by deep brain stimulation of the subthalamic nucleus

In studies implementing strict selection criteria in recruiting Parkinsonian patients for deep brain stimulation of the subthalamic nucleus, the prevalence of dementia was relatively low, even at long-term follow-up (Krack et al., 2003; Fasano et al., 2010).

In a 5-year follow-up study, the prevalence of dementia was 6%, as 3 out of 49 patients developed dementia 5 years after surgery (Krack et al., 2003).

In the cohort of Parkinsonian patients with 8-year follow-up mentioned above (Fasano et al., 2010), there was a 5% prevalence of dementia. In this latter study, 5 years after surgery only one out of 20 patients developed dementia, which had progressed at 8 years (Fasano et al., 2010). Such prevalence rates are lower than those reported in other studies investigating less strictly selected Parkinsonian patients, such as one study reporting in Parkinsonian patients a 38% prevalence of dementia after 10 years of follow-up (Hughes et al., 2000).

However, in one 3-year follow-up study carried out in 57 Parkinsonian patients treated by deep brain stimulation of the subthalamic nucleus (Aybek at al., 2007), dementia appeared in 5 out of 57 patients (8.7%) 6 months post surgery and in 24.5% of the patients 3 years post surgery, while the rest of the cohort remained cognitively stable over the whole follow-up. These Authors pointed out that in their cohort the prevalence of dementia over 3 years after deep brain stimulation of the subthalamic nucleus is similar to the prevalence reported in medically treated patients (Aybek at al., 2007). Moreover, in this cohort of patients treated by deep brain stimulation of the subthalamic nucleus some demographic and clinical variables (older age, presence of hallucinations, poorer performance on executive tasks) were preoperative risk factors of developing dementia (Aybek at al., 2007).

The observation of a relatively high prevalence (8.7%) of dementia 6 months post surgery may suggest the hypothesis that less strict selection criteria were employed in this study (Aybek at al., 2007), as compared with other studies with long-term follow-up reporting a lower incidence of dementia (Krack et al., 2003; Fasano et al., 2010).

2.6 Conclusive remarks on the effects deep brain stimulation of the subthalamic nucleus on cognition

Most neuropsychological studies in Parkinsonian patients treated by deep brain stimulation of the subthalamic nucleus share a methodological limitation, namely the lack of a control group of medically-treated Parkinsonian patients, which should be matched at baseline to patients who undergo deep brain stimulation of the subthalamic nucleus as to various clinical and demographic variables (age, educational level, overall cognitive status, severity of motor impairment).

Comparisons between Parkinsonian patients treated by deep brain stimulation of the subthalamic nucleus and medically treated Parkinsonian patients may allow to take into account cognitive decline due to aging and disease progression, particularly in patients with long-term follow-up.

However, in most studies which recruited a control group of medically-treated Parkinsonian patients the follow-up was relatively short, with follow-up periods of 6 months (Witt et al., 2008), 1 year (Castelli et al., 2010), 2 years (Williams et al., 2011) and 3 years (Zangaglia et al., 2009). Studies recruiting a control group of medically-treated Parkinsonian patients with a longer follow-up period are currently needed.

Only some neuropsychological investigations have attempted to discriminate between the effects on cognitive performance of the surgical intervention and the effects on cognitive performance of deep brain stimulation of the subthalamic nucleus itself (Jahanshahi et al., 2000; Pillon et al., 2000; Daniele et al., 2003), by comparing cognitive performance on neuropsychological tasks in different stimulation condition, namely with stimulators turned "ON" versus with stimulators turned "OFF".

In one study (Jahanshahi et al., 2000), performance on neuropsychological tasks of executive functions was investigated in 7 patients with Parkinson's disease treated by deep brain stimulation of the subthalamic nucleus and 6 patients treated by deep brain stimulation of the internal globus pallidus. Patients were assessed three times: with stimulators OFF, with stimulators ON, with stimulators OFF gain. With stimulators ON, in both groups of patients (Jahanshahi et al., 2000) there was a decline in a conditional associative learning task and an improved performance on several tasks assessing executive functions (Trail Making test part A and B, missing digit test, paced visual serial addition test, colour naming subtest of the Stroop Test). Moreover, with stimulators ON, only the subthalamic group showed a significant improvement on some additional tasks assessing executive functions (random number generation, Modified Wisconsin Card Sorting Test).

In another study (Pillon et al., 2000), cognitive performance of Parkinsonian patients treated by deep brain stimulation of either the subthalamic nucleus or the internal globus pallidus was assessed postoperatively at 3 months and 12 months, in different stimulation conditions. In this study, the group of patients treated by subthalamic implants showed in ON-stimulation condition an improved cognitive performance on neuropsychological tasks of psychomotor speed and spatial working memory (Pillon et al., 2000).

In patients with Parkinson's disease, the investigation of the effects on cognition of deep brain stimulation of the subthalamic nucleus as compared to the internal globus pallidus is of remarkable importance, in order to establish the potential beneficial and detrimental effects of both procedures.

In patients with Parkinson's disease who were treated by unilateral (Vingerhoets et al., 1999) or bilateral (Field et al., 1999) deep brain stimulation of the internal globus pallidus, preliminary short-term studies with a 3-month follow-up did not detect significant postoperative changes in cognitive performance.

By contrast, some investigations detected a mild decline on tasks of semantic verbal fluency (Volkmann et al., 2004) or executive dysfunction (Dujardin et al., 2000) in patients treated by bilateral deep brain stimulation of the internal globus pallidus and a mild decline on visuoconstructional tasks and on tasks of semantic verbal fluency in patients who underwent unilateral deep brain stimulation of the internal globus pallidus (Tröster et al., 1997).

A prospective randomized trial assessed cognition and mood in 23 patients treated by unilateral deep brain stimulation of the internal globus pallidus, as compared to 22 patients treated by unilateral deep brain stimulation of the subthalamic nucleus (Okun et al., 2009).

In this study, a significantly greater decline on a task of phonological verbal fluency was detected 7 months after surgery in the group who underwent subthalamic implants, as compared to the group treated by deep brain stimulation of the internal globus pallidus.

Moreover, in a multicenter long-term study carried out in 35 Parkinsonian patients treated by bilateral deep brain stimulation of the subthalamic nucleus and in 16 patients treated by bilateral deep brain stimulation of the internal globus pallidus (Moro et al., 2010), 5 to 6 years after surgery the occurrence of cognitive decline was higher in the group with subthalamic implants (23% of patients), as compared to the group with implants in the internal globus pallidus (12% of the patients).

In conclusion, although cognitive morbidity after deep brain stimulation of the subthalamic nucleus is relatively low, deep brain stimulation of the internal globus pallidus seems to have even a lower cognitive morbidity and might be a safer option in Parkinsonian patients who are more at risk for cognitive impairment.

3. Effects of deep brain stimulation of the subthalamic nucleus on behavioural symptoms

In Parkinsonian patients treated by deep brain stimulation of the subthalamic nucleus, both transient behavioural symptoms (apathy, manic symptoms, hypersexuality) and persistent behavioural symptoms (apathy, impulse control disorders, punding, depression with increased suicidal tendencies in some patients) have been described. On the other hand, some studies reported in Parkinsonian patients treated by subthalamic implants a postoperative improvement of behavioural symptoms (depression, anxiety, hallucinations, impulse control disorders).

3.1 Effects of deep brain stimulation of the subthalamic nucleus on mood

3.1.1 Depressive symptoms: Clinical presentation, evolution, and pathophysiology

After implants for deep brain stimulation of the subthalamic nucleus, some studies detected a postoperative improvement of depression (Daniele et al., 2003; Houeto et al., 2006; Kalteis et al., 2006) or no change in depressive symptoms (Drapier et al., 2006; York et al., 2008), while other studies reported the appearance or the worsening of depressive symptoms (Takeshita et al. 2005, Castelli et al., 2006; Temel et al. 2006).

In patients with Parkinson's disease treated by deep brain stimulation of the subthalamic nucleus, the proportion of subjects in which depressive symptoms appear or worsen after surgery as a persistent behavioural change varies between 2% up to 33%, according to different studies (Takeshita et al., 2005, Temel et al., 2006). Such appearance or worsening of depressive symptoms may be detected also in Parkinsonian patients who show a satisfactory postoperative improvement of motor symptoms.

A previously mentioned long-term follow-up study in 20 consecutive Parkinsonian patients who received by deep brain stimulation of the subthalamic nucleus (Fasano et al., 2010) did not detect any significant postoperative change on scales assessing depression 8 years after surgery, as compared with preoperative baseline.

In a previously mentioned prospective randomized study aimed at comparing mood in 22 patients treated by unilateral deep brain stimulation of the subthalamic nucleus and 23 patients treated by unilateral deep brain stimulation of the internal globus pallidus, 7 months after surgery changes in mood did not significantly differ between the two groups of patients (Okun et al., 2009).

In those Parkinsonian patients who show a postoperative improvement of depressive symptoms, such improvement has been interpreted as resulting either from a psychological response to the amelioration of Parkinsonian motor symptoms (Jahanshahi et al., 2000) or to the effects of deep brain stimulation of the subthalamic nucleus on neural systems which play a role in mood (Romito et al., 2002).

It has been hypothesized that in Parkinsonian patients treated with subthalamic implants postoperative depression might result either from the reduction of daily doses of dopaminergic drugs (Giovannoni et al, 2000) or from an indirect inhibition of the activity of serotonergic neurons in the dorsal raphe nuclei induced by deep brain stimulation of the subthalamic nucleus (Temel et al., 2007), possibly through various structures (ventral pallidum, substantia nigra pars reticulata, medial prefrontal cortex) which directly project to dorsal raphe nuclei (Tan et al., 2001).

3.1.2 Depressive symptoms: Treatment and prognosis

After deep brain stimulation of the subthalamic nucleus, suicidal tendencies have been reported in some Parkinsonian patients (Soulas et al., 2008; Voon et al., 2008).

In a retrospective survey carried out in 5311 Parkinsonian patients treated with subthalamic implants (Voon et al., 2008) the rate of completed suicide was 0.45%, while the rate of attempted suicide was 0.90%. In this study, an increased risk of attempted suicide was associated with a number of factors (postoperative depression, previous history of impulse control disorders or compulsive medication use, being single) and the highest rate of suicides was detected in the first postoperative year.

In another retrospective survey carried out in a smaller sample (n = 200) of Parkinsonian patients who underwent subthalamic implants (Soulas et al., 2008), despite a remarkable motor improvement, there was a higher than expected frequency of suicide (1% of completed suicide, 2% of attempted suicide) and suicidal behaviour was associated with postoperative depression and altered impulse control.

These latter studies (Soulas et al., 2008; Voon et al., 2008) show that there might be an increased risk of suicidal behaviour in Parkinsonian patients treated with subthalamic implants, suggesting that the main risk factor for attempted and completed suicide is postsurgical depression, which on postoperative follow-up should be adequately diagnosed and treated with anti-depressant drugs.

3.1.3 Manic symptoms: Clinical presentation, evolution, and pathophysiology

A systematic review of a large sample (n = 1398) of Parkinsonian patients who underwent bilateral brain stimulation of the subthalamic nucleus showed that the occurrence of manic symptoms was reported in about 4% of PD patients (Temel et al., 2006), more frequently early after surgery (Romito et al., 2002; Schupbach et al., 2005; Visser-Vandewalle et al., 2005; Contarino et al., 2007).

Manic symptoms in patients treated by subthalamic implants mostly last few hours or few days and are usually observed after stimulation of contacts in the ventral part of the substantia nigra, probably in the substantia nigra pars reticulata (Ulla et al., 2006; Ulla et al., 2011).

In some patients, however, manic symptoms might be induced by stimulation of contacts within the subthalamic nucleus (Ulla et al., 2011; Mallet et al., 2007), especially by stimulation of a ventral contact of the electrode within the subthalamic nucleus. In these cases, manic symptoms may disappear by switching off this ventral contact (Mallet et al. 2007). It has been also suggested that stimulation of axons projecting from medial (limbic) subthalamic nucleus to the medial forebrain bundle might give rise to transient reversible hypomania (Coenen et al., 2009).

In Parkinsonian patients who show stimulation-induced manic symptoms after subthalamic implants (Ulla et al., 2011), positron emission tomography showed during the manic state an increase of regional cerebral blood flow in various structures (anterior cingulate cortex, the medial prefrontal cortex, primary motor cortex, globus pallidus), mainly in the right cerebral hemisphere.

These findings support the hypothesis that a dysfunction of limbic structures (particularly, the anterior cingulate cortex and the medial prefrontal cortex) in the right cerebral hemisphere, induced by stimulation of the substantia nigra or the subthalamic nucleus, might play a critical role in the pathophysiology of manic states induced by subthalamic implants in Parkinsonian patients.

3.1.4 Manic symptoms: Treatment and prognosis

In Parkinsonian patients, manic symptoms may disappear after switching to other targets to be stimulated (Raucher-Chene et al., 2008) or readjusting the parameters of stimulation (Mandat et al., 2006).

3.2 Effects of deep brain stimulation of the subthalamic nucleus on apathy

3.2.1 Apathy: Clinical presentation, evolution, and pathophysiology

Apathy, which may be defined as loss of motivation (Marin, 1991), is a common behavioural symptom in patients with Parkinson's disease.

Most studies assessing apathy before and after surgery in Parkinsonian patients treated by subthalamic implants found a postoperative worsening of apathy (Funkiewiez et al., 2004; Schupbach et al., 2005; Drapier et al., 2006; Contarino et al., 2007; Le Jeune et al., 2009; Porat et al., 2009; Thobois et al., 2010), while two studies found no postoperative change in apathy (Castelli et al., 2006; Castelli et al., 2007). By contrast, in Parkinsonian patients who underwent bilateral deep brain stimulation of the subthalamic nucleus a transient improvement of apathy was detected after acute subthalamic stimulation, namely in ON stimulation as compared to OFF stimulation condition (Czernecki et al., 2005). To our knowledge, no study reported in Parkinsonian patients a significant improvement of chronic apathy following subthalamic implants.

It has been reported that after subthalamic implants a postoperative worsening of apathy may occur in the absence of significant postoperative changes of depression or anxiety (Drapier et al., 2006).

In a recent study (Kirsh-Darrow et al., 2011), apathy was assessed in Parkinsonian patients who underwent either unilateral deep brain stimulation of the internal globus pallidus (n = 15) or unilateral deep brain stimulation of the subthalamic nucleus (n = 33) and in a control group of medically treated Parkinsonian patients (n = 48). The results of this study show that apathy progressively increased up to 6 months after both subthalamic and pallidal unilateral implants, while it was unchanged in the non-surgical group of Parkinsonian patients (Kirsh-Darrow et al., 2011). In this study, the degree of apathy in patients who underwent deep brain stimulation was not related to postsurgical changes in levodopa equivalent daily doses (Kirsh-Darrow et al., 2011).

In a prospective study focused on the occurrence of apathy and associated symptoms in 63 patients with Parkinson's disease treated with deep brain stimulation of the subthalamic nucleus (Thobois et al., 2010), apathy appeared in 34 patients after a mean of 4.7 months and was reversible in 17 patients by the 12-month follow-up.

In this study, [11C]-raclopride positron emission tomography showed that binding values were greater in apathetic Parkinsonian patients in various structures (orbitofrontal, dorsolateral prefrontal, posterior cingulate and temporal cortices, left striatum and right amygdala) bilaterally, suggesting a greater dopamine D2/D3 receptor density or reduced synaptic dopamine level in such structures.

3.2.2 Apathy: Treatment and prognosis

The effects of a 6-week treatment with the dopamine D2-D3 agonist ropinirole was investigated in 8 Parkinsonian patients who developed apathy after complete withdrawal from dopaminergic medication, following successful subthalamic implants (Czernecki et al., 2008). In 7 out of 8 Parkinsonian patients (in which the stimulation contacts were located within the subthalamic nucleus), ropinirole induced an improvement of apathy, while only one patient (in whom the stimulation contacts were located within the zona incerta) remained apathetic. This study suggests that in Parkinsonian patients treated by subthalamic implants apathy may result from a dopaminergic deficiency in associative limbic areas and can be effectively treated in most patients by dopaminergic agonists administered postoperatively (Czernecki et al., 2008).

3.3 Effects of deep brain stimulation of the subthalamic nucleus on anxiety

3.3.1 Anxiety: Clinical presentation, evolution, and pathophysiology

After subthalamic implants, a number of studies showed in Parkinsonian patients a postoperative improvement of anxiety (Daniele et al., 2003; Houeto et al., 2006; Kalteis et al., 2006; Schupbach et al., 2007) or no change in anxiety symptoms (Drapier et al. , 2006; York et al., 2008), while other studies reported the appearance or the worsening of anxiety (Rodriguez-Oroz et al. 2005; Castelli et al., 2006).

The postoperative improvement of anxiety observed in some studies might result from the beneficial effects of subthalamic implants on the motor symptoms of Parkinson'disease (Daniele et al., 2003).

On the other hand, in Parkinsonian patients treated by subthalamic implants, in which a marked reduction of daily doses of dopaminergic drugs is usually obtained postoperatively, it has been hypothesized that a postoperative worsening of anxiety might result from a delayed dopamine withdrawal syndrome (Thobois et al., 2010).

In Parkinsonian patients, individual differences in both dopaminergic treatment and in the extent of denervation of dopaminergic mesolimbic systems might explain the variable effects of deep brain stimulation of the subthalamic nucleus on anxiety, mood and motivation/apathy (Thobois et al., 2010).

3.3.2 Anxiety: Treatment and prognosis

So far, the issue of treatment of anxiety symptoms in Parkinsonian patients who undergo subthalamic implants has been poorly investigated.

In a study with a 6-month follow-up period in which patients were randomly assigned to have subthalamic implants (n = 63) or the best medical treatment for Parkinson's disease (n = 60), anxiety was reduced in the subthalamic implant group, as compared with the medically-treated group (Witt et al., 2008). In a long-term follow-up study in 20 Parkinsonian patients who received subthalamic implants, 8 years after surgery no significant change was observed on a scale assessing anxiety, as compared with baseline (Fasano et al., 2010).

3.4 Effects of deep brain stimulation of the subthalamic nucleus on psychotic symptoms

3.4.1 Psychotic symptoms: Clinical presentation, evolution, and pathophysiology

In Parkinsonian patients treated by bilateral subthalamic implants, hallucinations and delusions may appear as transient behavioural symptoms shortly after surgery (Romito et al., 2002).

It is still matter of debate whether Parkinsonian patients with history of hallucination may be good candidates for subthalamic implants.

A retrospective review of 10 Parkinsonian patients who suffered from severe medication-induced hallucinations or delusions and underwent bilateral subthalamic implants (Umemura et al., 2011) showed that such psychotic symptoms disappeared in 8 out of 10 patients after postoperative reduction of dopaminergic medication. By contrast, in 2 out of 10 patients hallucinations and delusions worsened immediately after surgery (despite complete withdrawal of dopaminergic medication), but disappeared after treatment with anti-psychotic drugs for some months (Umemura et al., 2011). On the whole, such retrospective review suggests that deep brain stimulation of the subthalamic nucleus is a good treatment option in Parkinsonian patients with medication-induced hallucinations or delusions, provided that the possible worsening of psychotic symptoms which may be observed in a subgroup of patients is carefully monitored and treated.

In a further study aimed at assessing the effects of subthalamic implants on preexisting hallucinations in 18 patients with advanced Parkinson's disease (Yoshida et al., 2009), six months after the implant there was a significant postoperative improvement of severity of hallucinations, as compared with baseline.

These latter studies (Umemura et al., 2011; Yoshida et al., 2009) suggest that in patients with advanced Parkinson's disease a history of hallucinations is not a contraindication to subthalamic implants.

In conclusion, it might be hypothesized that in most Parkinsonian patients with medication-induced hallucinations a postoperative reduction of dopaminergic anti-Parkinsonian drugs might play a critical role in the postoperative improvement of hallucinations.

3.4.2 Psychotic symptoms: Treatment and prognosis

As mentioned above, treatment with anti-psychotic drugs is indicated in Parkinsonian patients in whom hallucinations and delusions worsen immediately after surgery (Umemura et al., 2011). In a group of Parkinsonian patients followed up for 3 years after deep brain stimulation of the subthalamic nucleus, the use of antipsychotic drugs was stable until 1 year, while there was a subsequent increase in the use of antipsychotic drugs at 3 years (Zibetti et al., 2009).

3.5 Effects of deep brain stimulation of the subthalamic nucleus on impulse control disorders

3.5.1 Impulse control disorders: Clinical presentation, evolution, and pathophysiology

In Parkinsonian patients treated by deep brain stimulation of the subthalamic nucleus, impulse control disorders (pathological gambling, hypersexuality, compulsive eating and buying/shopping) may occasionally appear after surgery, while in most cases preexisting impulse control disorders may improve or disappear after subthalamic implants (Broen et al., 2011; Witjas et al., 2005; Bandini et al., 2007; Ardouin et al., 2006; Lim et al., 2009).

As to pathological gambling (Lim et al., 2009) and hypersexuality (Doshi & Bargava, 2008), these disorders may be occasionally be observed in some Parkinsonian patients after subthalamic implants, while Parkinsonian patients may rarely develop compulsive eating after subthalamic implants (Zahodne et al., 2011). A weight gain, which may result from multiple pathogenic factors besides compulsive eating, may be detected in up 48% of Parkinsonian patients after deep brain stimulation of the subthalamic nucleus (Piboolnurak et al., 2007).

In Parkinsonian patients who show a postoperative improvement of preexisting impulse control disorders, such improvement might be due to at least two mechanisms. The most plausible mechanism is a reduction of dopaminergic medication after the subthalamic implants, which leads to decreased stimulation of mesolimbic dopaminergic circuits (Ardouin et al., 2006). Alternatively, it has been proposed that deep brain stimulation of the subthalamic nucleus may induce inhibitory effects on dopaminergic and serotoninergic pathways ascending to limbic circuits involved in reward (Witjas et al., 2005).

On the other hand, in some Parkinsonian patients, impulse control disorders appear after subthalamic implants, notwithstanding with a postoperative reduction of doses of dopaminergic drugs (Romito et al., 2002; Doshi and Bargava, 2008; Smeding et al., 2007; Sensi et al., 2004; Lim et al., 2009). In these latter patients, it might be hypothesised that deep brain stimulation of the subthalamic nucleus may induce changes in the activity of limbic circuits involving the subthalamic nucleus or involving fibres adjacent to this nucleus, giving rise to a tendency to impulsivity (Demetriades et al, 2011). A neurophysiological study aimed at recording local field potentials in the subthalamic nucleus of Parkinsonian patients patients treated by deep brain stimulation of the subthalamic nucleus (Rodriguez-Oroz et al., 2011) showed an oscillatory theta-alpha activity in the ventral subthalamic nucleus, which was associated with impulse control disorders, suggesting that such limbic ventral subthalamic area might be involved in the development of impulse control disorders in these Parkinsonian patients.

It has been previously mentioned that the subthalamic nucleus and prefrontal cortical areas might play a critical role in decision-making processes and that patients with Parkinson's disease may show after deep brain stimulation of the subthalamic nucleus a reduced ability to slow down their decisions in high-conflict conditions, resulting in increased impulsivity (Frank et al., 2007).

3.5.2 Impulse control disorders: Treatment and prognosis

In a cross-sectional study aimed at comparing Parkinsonian patients treated by subthalamic implants versus Parkinsonian patients treated by anti-Parkinsonian drugs but eligible for deep brain stimulation (Halbig et al. , 2009), impulsivity was assessed by the Barratt Impulsiveness Scale and was higher in patients with subthalamic implants. In this study, the prevalence of impulse control disorders was higher (3 out of 16 subjects, namely 19%) in patients treated by subthalamic implants than in medically treated Parkinsonian patients (3 out of 37 subjects, namely 8%). The Authors suggest that screening for impulsivity and impulse control disorders should be performed prior to deep brain stimulation (Halbig et al. , 2009).

In conclusion, since the effects of brain stimulation of the subthalamic nucleus on impulse control disorders in Parkinsonian patients are variable, the prognosis of such disorders may vary from patient to patient, although in most Parkinsonian patients preexisting impulse control disorders may improve or disappear after subthalamic implants. Further studies are needed in order to clarify the issue of treatment strategies in those patients in whom impulse control disorders do appear or worsen after surgery.

3.6 Long-term behavioural follow-up in patients treated by deep brain stimulation of the subthalamic nucleus

In the previously mentioned study assessing motor and cognitive outcome in patients with Parkinson's disease 8 years after subthalamic implants (Fasano et al., 2010), in the overall group of patients there was no significant change 8 years after surgery on behavioural scales assessing depression and anxiety, as compared to preoperative baseline. In the cohort of 20 Parkinsonian patients who completed the 8-year follow-up (Fasano et al., 2010), a number of persistent behavioral adverse events were reported, such as depressive symptoms (in 25% of the patients), apathy (in 20% of the patients), psychotic symptoms (in 20% of the patients), hypersexuality (in 5% of the patients).

3.7 An explicative case of a Parkinsonian patient with manic symptoms after bilateral subthalamic implants

A 52-year-old right-handed man presented a 11-year history of severe rigid–akinetic Parkinson's disease, which became poorly responsive to anti-Parkinsonian medication (Romito et al., 2002). This patient, who had a family history of major depression, at the age of 26 years suffered from a major depressive episode, during his father's terminal illness.

The patient received a implant of quadripolar leads bilaterally in the subthalamic nucleus under stereotactic guidance. Compared to preoperative assessment, he showed a marked improvement of Parkinsonian motor symptoms and activities of daily living, while wearing-off phenomena and on-state dyskinesias (reported before the implantation) disappeared.

Two days after the implant, the patient developed a manic syndrome (Romito et al., 2002), characterized by inflated self-esteem and grandiosity, marked increase in goal-directed activities, need to purchase unneeded items, decreased need for sleep, planning of hazardous business investments, flights of ideas. His appetite decreased and the patient lost 5 to 6 kg. Sexual desire and sexual activity increased and the patient had frequent spontaneous erections, although he was not on dopamine agonists. Despite a lack of interest in religion, he started to spend much time in writing poems on religious themes. Moreover, the patient became irritable, litigious, and over-reactive. A diagnosis of manic episode was made.

When the stimulator was turned off, there was a rapid worsening of Parkinsonian motor symptoms but manic symptoms did not improve (Romito et al., 2002).

In this patient, all antiparkinsonian medication was discontinued 1 month after surgery. Stimulation settings remained unchanged from the second month on. During postoperative follow-up up to 12 months after surgery, he showed no significant change in cognitive performance on neuropsychological tasks, as compared to preoperative performance.

In agreement with his wife, the patient was followed up very carefully, but no pharmacological treatment for manic symptoms was prescribed. Three months after their onset, manic symptoms gradually decreased and then disappeared completely. Twelve months after the subthalamic implant, the patient showed a slight reduction of initiative, in the absence of any significant impairment in daily living activities (Romito et al., 2002).

4. Conclusions

Cognitive and behavioural disturbances in patients with Parkinson's disease seem to be relatively more frequent after deep brain stimulation of the subthalamic nucleus, as compared with deep brain stimulation of the internal globus pallidus. This finding might be at least partially due to the fact that the subthalamic nucleus is a smaller target, with different neural circuits (motor, associative, and limbic circuits) in close proximity to each other. Thus, electrode misplacements or current spreading to non-motor circuits involving the subthalamic nucleus may give rise to cognitive and behavioural disturbances after subthalamic implants.

On the whole, nonetheless, most studies agree about the view that the cognitive and behavioural morbidity of deep brain stimulation of the subthalamic nucleus in patients with Parkinson's disease can be considered relatively low, even in the long term, provided that appropriate criteria are used to select candidates for neurosurgery,

Further studies are certainly needed to elucidate the pathophysiological mechanisms underlying the postoperative cognitive and behavioural changes which may be observed in Parkinsonian patients treated by deep brain stimulation of the subthalamic nucleus.

5. References

Aarsland D., Brønnick K., Alves G. et al. (2009). The spectrum of neuropsychiatric symptoms in patients with early untreated Parkinson's disease. *Journal of Neurology, Neurosurgery and Psychiatry*, Vol.80, pp. 928-930

Alegret M., Junque C., Valldeoriola F. et al. (2001). Effects of bilateral subthalamic stimulation on cognitive function in Parkinson disease. *Archives of Neurology,* Vol.58, pp. 1223–7

Alexander G.E., De Long M.R.& Strick P.L. (1986). Parallel organization of functionally segregated circuits linking basal ganglia and cortex. *Annual Review of Neuroscience,* Vol.9, pp. 357-381

Ambermoon P., Carter A., Hall W. et al. (2011). Compulsive use of dopamine replacement therapy: a model for stimulant drug addiction? *Addiction.* Vol.106, pp. 283-293

Ardouin C., Pillon B., Peiffer E. et al. (1999). Bilateral subthalamic or pallidal stimulationfor Parkinson's disease affects neither memory nor executive functions: a consecutive series of 62 patients. *Annals of Neurology,* Vol.46, pp 217–23

Ardouin C., Voon V., Worbe Y. et al. (2006). Pathological gambling in Parkinson's disease improves on chronic subthalamic nucleus stimulation. *Movement Disorders* Vol.2, No.11, pp. 1941-6

Aybek S., Gronchi-Perrin A., Berney A. et al. (2009). Long-term cognitive profile and incidence of dementia after STN-DBS in Parkinson's disease. *Movement Disorders,* Vol.15, No.22(7), pp. 974-81

Bandini F., Primavera A., Pizzorno M., & Cocito L. (2007). Using STN DBS and medication reduction as a strategy to treat pathological gambling in Parkinson's disease. *Parkinsonism Related Disorders,* Vol.13, No.6, pp. 369-71

Boller F, Passafiume D, Keefe NC et al. (1984). Visuospatial impairment in Parkinson's disease. Role of perceptual and motor factors. *Archives of Neurology,* Vol.41, pp. 485-490

Braak H., Ghebremedhin E., Rub U. et al. (2004). Stages in the development of Parkinson's disease-related pathology. *Cell Tissue Research,* Vol.318, pp. 121-134

Broen M., Duits A., Visser-Vandewalle V. et al. (2011). Impulse control and related disorders in Parkinson's disease patients treated with bilateral subthalamic nucleus stimulation: A review. *Parkinsonism Related Disorders.* Vol.17, No.6, pp. 413-7

Bugalho P., da Silva J.A., Cargaleiro I. et al. (2012, in press). Psychiatric symptoms screening in the early stages of Parkinson's disease. *Journal of Neurology.* DOI 10.1007/s00415-011-6140-8

Burn D.J. (2002). Beyond the Iron mask: towards better recognition and treatment of depression associated with Parkinson's disease. *Movement Disorders,* Vol.17, pp. 445-454

Candy J.M., Perry R.H., Perry E.K. et al. (1983). Pathological changes in the nucleus of Meynert in Alzheimer's and Parkinson's disease. *Journal of Neurological Sciences* Vol.59, pp. 277-289

Cash R., Dennis T., L'Hereux R. et al (1987). Parkinson's disease and dementia: norepinephrine and dopamine in locus coeruleus. *Neurology* Vol.37, pp. 42-46

Castelli L., Perozzo P., Zibetti M. et al. (2006). Chronic deep brain stimulation of the subthalamic nucleus for Parkinson's disease: effects on cognition, mood, anxiety and personality traits.*European Neurology* Vol.55, No.3, pp. 136-144

Castelli L., Lanotte M., Zibetti M. et al. (2007). Apathy and verbal fluency in STN-stimulated PD patients. An observational follow-up study. *Journal of Neurology*, Vol. 254, No.9, pp. 1238-1243

Castelli L., Rizzi L., Zibetti M. et al. (2010). Neuropsychological changes 1-year after subthalamic DBS in PD patients: A prospective controlled study. *Parkinsonism Related Disorders*, Vol.16, No2, pp. 115-8

Coenen, V.A., Honey C.R., Hurwitz T. et al. (2009). Medial forebrain bundle stimulation as a pathophysiological mechanism for hypomania in subthalamic nucleus deep brain stimulation for Parkinson's disease. *Neurosurgery*, Vol.64, No.6, pp. 1106-1114; discussion 1114-1105

Contarino M. F., Daniele A., Sibilia A.H. et al. (2007). Cognitive outcome 5 years after bilateral chronic stimulation of subthalamic nucleus in patients with Parkinson's disease. *Journal of Neurology, Neurosurgery and Psychiatry*, Vol.78, No.3, pp. 248-252

Cools R., Barker R.A., Sahakian B.J. & Robbins T.W. (2001). Mechanism of cognitive set flexibility in Parkinson's disease. *Brain*, Vol.124, pp. 2503-2512

Cooper J.A., Sagar H.J., Jordan N. et al. (1991). Cognitive impairment in early untreated Parkinson's disease and its relationship to motor disability. *Brain*, Vol.114, pp. 2095-2122

Cubo E., Bernard B., Leurgans S. et al. (2000). Cognitive and motor functions in patients with Parkinson's disease with and without depression. *Clinical Neuropharmacology*, Vol.23, No.6, pp. 331-334

Czernecki V., Pillon B., Houeto J.L. et al. (2005). Does bilateral stimulation of the subthalamic nucleus aggravate apathy in Parkinson's disease?, *Journal of Neurology, Neurosurgery and Psychiatry*, Vol.76, No.6, pp. 775-779

Czernecki V., Schüpbach M., Yaici S. et al. (2008). Apathy following subthalamic stimulation in Parkinson disease: a dopamine responsive symptom. *Movement Disorders*, Vol.23, No.7, pp. 964-969

Daniele A., Albanese A., Contarino M.F. et al. (2003). Cognitive and behavioural effects of chronic stimulation of the subthalamic nucleus in patients with Parkinson's disease. *Journal of Neurology, Neurosurgery and Psychiatry*, Vol.74, pp. 175–82

Demetriades P., Rickards H. & Cavanna A.E. (2011). Impulse control disorders following deep brain stimulation of the subthalamic nucleus in Parkinson's disease: clinical aspects. *Parkinson's disease.* doi:10.4061/2011/658415

Doshi P. & Bhargava P. (2008). Hypersexuality following subthalamic nucleus stimulation for Parkinson's disease. *Neurology India*, Vol.56, No.4, pp. 474-476

Drapier D., Drapier S., Sauleau P. et al. (2006). Does subthalamic nucleus stimulation induce apathy in Parkinson's disease? *Journal of Neurology* Vol.253, No. 8, pp. 1083-1091

Dubois & Pillon (1997). Cognitive deficits in Parkinson's disease. *Journal of Neurology*, Vol.244, pp. 2-8.

Dujardin K., Krystkowiak P., Defebvre L. et al. (2000). A case of severe dysexecutive syndrome consecutive to chronic bilateral pallidal stimulation. *Neuropsychologia.*, Vol. 38, No.9, pp. 1305-15

Dujardin K. Krystkowiak P., Defebvre L. et al (2001). Memory and executive function in sporadic and familial Parkinson's disease. *Brain.* Vol.124(Pt 2), pp. 389-98

Factor S.A., Mohlo E.S., Podskalny G.D. & Brown D. (1995). Parkinson's disease drug-induced psychiatric states. *Advances in Neurology*, Vol. 65, pp. 115-138

Fasano A., Romito L.M., Daniele A. et al. (2010). Motor and cognitive outcome in patients with Parkinson's disease 8 years after subthalamic implants. *Brain*, Vol.133, No.9, pp. 2664-76

Fields J.A., Tröster A.I., Wilkinson S.B. et al. (1999). Cognitive outcome following staged bilateral pallidal stimulation for the treatment of Parkinson's disease. *Clinical Neurology and Neurosurgery*, Vol. 101, No3, pp. 182-8

Frank M.J., Samanta J., Moustafa A.A. et al. (2007). Hold your horses: impulsivity, deep brain stimulation, and medication in parkinsonism. *Science*. Vol. 23, No.318, pp. 1309-12

Funkiewiez A., Ardouin C., Caputo E. et al. (2004). Long term effects of bilateral subthalamic nucleus stimulation on cognitive function, mood, and behaviour in Parkinson's disease. *Journal of Neurology, Neurosurgery and Psychiatry*, Vol.75, pp. 834-9

Giovannoni G., O' Sullivan J.D., Turner K., et al. (2000). Hedonistic homeostatic dysregulation in patients with Parkinson's disease on dopamine replacement therapies. *Journal of Neurology, Neurosurgery and Psychiatry*, Vol.68, No.4, pp. 423-8

Gotham A.M., Brown R.G. & Marsden C.D.(1986). Depression in Parkinson's Disease: a quantitative and qualitative analysis. *Journal of Neurology, Neurosurgery and Psychiatry*, Vol.49, No.4, pp. 381-389

Green J., McDonald W.M., Vitek J.L. et al. (2002). Cognitive impairment in advanced PD without dementia. *Neurology*, Vol. 59, pp. 1320-1324

Hälbig T.D., Tse W., Frisina P.G. et al. (2009). Subthalamic deep brain stimulation and impulse control in Parkinson's disease. *European Journal of Neurology*, Vol.16, No.4, pp. 493-7

Hamani C., Richter E., Schwalb J.M. et al. (2005). Bilateral subthalamic nucleus stimulation for Parkinson's disease: a systematic review of the clinical literature. *Neurosurgery*, Vol.56, No.6, pp.1313-21

Harrington D.L., Haaland K.Y., Yeo R.A. & Marder E. (1990). Procedural memory in Parkinson's disease. Impaired motor but not visuoperceptual learning. *Journal of Clinical and Experimental Neuropsychology*, Vol.12, pp. 223-239

Helkala E.L., Laulumaa V., Soininen H. & Riekkinen P.J. (1988). Recall and recognition memory in patients with Alzheimer's and Parkinson's diseases. *Annals of Neurology*, Vol.24, pp. 214-217

Houeto J.L., Mallet L., Mesnage V. et al. (2006). Subthalamic stimulation in Parkinson disease: behavior and social adaptation. *Archives of Neurology*, Vol.63, No.8, pp. 1090-5

Hoverstadt A., de Jong G.J., Meerwaldt J.D. et al. (1987). Spatial disorientation as an early symptom of Parkinson's disease. *Neurology*, Vol. 37, pp. 485-487

Hughes A.J., Daniel S.E. & Lees A.J. (1993). The clinical features of Parkinson's disease in 100 histologically proven cases. *Advances in Neurology*, Vol.60, pp. 595-9

Hughes T.A., Ross H.F., Musa S. et al. (2000). A 10-year study of the incidence of and factors predicting dementia in Parkinson's disease. *Neurology*, Vol.25, No.54(8), pp. 1596-1602

Jahanshahi M., Ardouin C.M., Brown R.G. et al. (2000). The impact of deep brain stimulation on executive function in Parkinson's disease. *Brain*, Vol.123 (Pt 6), pp. 1142-54

Kalteis K.H., Standhardt H., Kryspin-Exner I. et al. (2006). Influence of bilateral STN-stimulation on psychiatric symptoms and psychosocial functioning in patients with Parkinson's disease. *Journal of Neural Transmission*, Vol.113, No.9, pp. 1191-1206

Katzen, H., Myerson C., Papapetropoulos S., et al. (2010). Multi-modal hallucinations and cognitive function in Parkinson's disease.*Dementia and Geriatric Cognitive Disorders*, Vol. 30, No.1, pp. 51-56

Kirsch-Darrow L., Zahodne L.B., Marsiske M. et al. (2011). The trajectory of apathy after deep brain stimulation: from pre-surgery to 6 months post-surgery in Parkinson's disease. *Parkinsonism Related Disorders*, Vol.17, No.3, pp. 182-188

Krack P., Batir A., Van Blercom N. et al. (2003). Five-year follow-up of bilateral stimulation of the subthalamic nucleus in advanced Parkinson's disease. *New England Journal of Medicine*, Vol.349, pp. 1925–34

Kulisesky J., Avila A., Barbanoj M. et al. (1996). Acute effects of levodopa on neuropsychological performance in stable and fluctuating Parkinson's disease patients at different levodopa plasma levels. *Brain*, Vol.119, pp. 2121-2132

Leentjens A.F., Dujardin K., Marsh L., et al. (2008). Apathy and anhedonia rating scales in Parkinson's disease: critique and recommendation. *Movement Disorders*, Vol.23, pp. 2004-2014

Le Jeune F., Drapier D., Bourguignon A. et al. (2009). Subthalamic nucleus stimulation in Parkinson disease induces apathy: a PET study. *Neurology*, Vol.73, No.21, pp. 1746-1751

Lim S.Y., O'Sullivan S.S., Kotschet K. et al. (2009). Dopamine dysregulation syndrome, impulse control disorders and punding after deep brain stimulation surgery for Parkinson's disease. *Journal of Clinical Neuroscience*, Vol.16, No.9, pp. 1148-52

Litvan I., Mohr E., Williams J. et al. (1991). Differential memory and executive functions in demented patients with Parkinson's disease and Alzheimer's disease. *Journal of Neurology, Neurosurgery and Psychiatry*, Vol. 54, pp. 25-29

Malapani C., Pillon B., Dubois B. & Agid Y. (1994). Impaired simultaneous cognitive task performance in Parkinson's disease: a dopamine-related dysfunction. *Neurology*, Vol. 44, pp. 319-326

Mallet L., Schüpbach M., N'Diaye K. et al. (2007). Stimulation of subterritories of the subthalamic nucleus reveals its role in the integration of the emotional and motor aspects of behavior. *Proceedings of the National Academy of Sciences of the United States of America*, Vol.104, No25, pp. 10661-10666

Mandat, T. S., Hurwitz T. & Honey C.R. (2006). Hypomania as an adverse effect of subthalamic nucleus stimulation: report of two cases. *Acta Neurochirurgica (Wien)*, Vol.148, No.8, pp. 895-897

Marin R.S. (1991). Apathy: a neuropsychiatric syndrome. *Journal of Neuropsychiatry and Clinical Neurosciences*. Vol.3, No.3, pp.243-54

Marsh L. (2000). Neuropsychiatric aspects of Parkinson's disease. *Psychosomatics*, Vol.41, pp. 15-23

Matison R., Mayeux R., Rosen J. & Fahn S.(1982). "Tip-of-the-tongue" phenomenon in Parkinson's disease. *Neurology*, Vol. 32, pp. 567-570.

Mattay V.S., Tessitore A., Callicot J.H. et al. (2002). Dopaminergic modulation of cortical function in patients with Parkinson's disease. *Annals of Neurology* Vol.51, pp. 156-164

Mayberg H.S. & Solomon D.H. (1995). Depression in Parkinson's disease: a biochemical and organic viewpoint. In: *Behavioral neurology of movement disorders*, Weiner WJ, Lang AE (eds), Advances in Neurology Vol. 65. Raven Press Ltd, New York

Mayeux R., Stern Y., Sano M. et al. (1988). An estimate of the the prevalence of dementia in idiopathic Parkinson's disease. *Archives of Neurology*, Vol.45, pp. 260-262

Menza M., Dobkin R.D., Marin H. et al. (2009). The impact of treatment of depression on quality of life, disability and relapse in patients with Parkinson's disease. *Movement disorders* Vol.24, pp. 1325-1332

Mohr E., Litvan I., Williams J. et al. (1990). Selective deficits in Alzheimer and Parkinsonian dementia: visuospatial function. *Canadian Journal of neurological Sciences*, Vol.17, pp. 292-297

Mohr E., Mendis T. & Grimes J.D. (1995). Late cognitive changes in Parkinson's disease with an emphasis on dementia. In: *Behavioral neurology of movement disorders*, Weiner WJ, Lang AE (eds), Advances in Neurology Vol. 65. Raven Press Ltd, New York

Moro E., Lozano A.M., Pollak P. et al. (2010). Long-term results of a multicenter study on subthalamic and pallidal stimulation in Parkinson's disease. *Movement Disorders*, Vol.25, No5, pp.578-86

Morris R.G., Downes J.J., Sahakian B.J. et al. (1988). Planning and spatial working memory in Parkinson's disease. *Journal of Neurology, Neurosurgery and Psychiatry*, Vol. 135, pp. 669-675

Okun M.S., Fernandez H.H., Wu S.S. et al. (2009). Cognition and mood in Parkinson's disease in subthalamic nucleus versus globus pallidus interna deep brain stimulation: the COMPARE trial. *Annals of Neurology*, Vol.65, No.5, pp. 586-9

Parsons T.D., Rogers S.A., Braaten A.J. et al. (2006). Cognitive sequelae of subthalamic nucleus deep brain stimulation in Parkinson's disease: a meta-analysis. *Lancet Neurology*, Vol.5, No.7, pp. 578-88

Paulus W. & Jellinger K. (1991). The neuropathologic basis of different clinical subgroups of Parkinson's disease. *Journal of Neuropathology and Experimental Neurology*, Vol.50, pp. 743-755

Pedersen K.F., Larsen J.P., Alves G. et al. (2009). Prevalence and clinical correlates of apathy in Parkinson's disease: a community-based study. *Parkinsonism and Related Disorders*, Vol.15, pp. 295-299

Péran P., Rascol O., Démonet J.F. et al. (2003). Deficit of verb generation in nondemented patients with Parkinson's disease. *Movement Disorders*, Vol.18, No.2, pp. 150-6.

Piboolnurak P., Lang A.E., Lozano A.M. et al. (2007). Levodopa response in long-term bilateral subthalamic stimulation for Parkinson's disease. *Movement Disorders*, Vol.22, No.7, pp. 990-7

Pillon B., Ardouin C., Damier P. et al. (2000). Neuropsychological changes between "off"and "on" STN or GPi stimulation in Parkinson's disease. *Neurology*, Vol. 55, pp. 411–18

Porat O., Cohen O.S., Schwartz R. et al. (2009). Association of preoperative symptom profile with psychiatric symptoms following subthalamic nucleus stimulation in patients with Parkinson's disease. *Journal of Neuropsychiatry and Clinical Neurosciences*, Vol. 21, No.4, pp. 398-405

Ransmayr G., Schmidhuber-Eiler B., Karamat E. et al. (1987). Visuoperception and visuospatial and visuorotational performance in Parkinson's disease. *Journal of Neurology*, Vol. 235, pp. 99-101

Raucher-Chene D., Charrel C. L., de Maindreville A.D. et al. (2008). Manic episode with psychotic symptoms in a patient with Parkinson's disease treated by subthalamic nucleus stimulation: improvement on switching the target. *Journal of Neurological Sciences*, Vol. 273(1-2), pp. 116-117

Robbins T.W., James M., Owen A.M. et al. (1994). Cognitive deficits in progressive sopranuclear palsy. Parkinson's disease and multiple system atrophy in tests sensitive to frontal lobe dysfunction. *Journal of Neurology, Neurosurgery and Psychiatry*, Vol. 57, pp. 79-88

Rodriguez-Oroz M.C., Obeso J.A., Lang A.E. et al. (2005). Bilateral deep brain stimulation in Parkinson's disease: a multicentre study with 4 years follow-up. *Brain*, Vol. 128 (Pt 10), pp. 2240-9

Rodriguez-Oroz M. C., Lopez-Azcarate J., Garcia-Garcia D. et al. (2011). Involvement of the subthalamic nucleus in impulse control disorders associated with Parkinson's disease. *Brain*, Vol.134 (Pt 1), pp. 36-49

Romito L.M., Raja M., Daniele A. et al. (2002). Transient mania with hypersexuality after surgery for high frequency stimulation of the subthalamic nucleus in Parkinson's disease. *Movement Disorders*, Vol. 17, No.6, pp. 1371-4

Saint-Cyr J.A., Trépanier L.L., Kumar R. et al. (2000). Neuropsychological consequences of chronic bilateral stimulation of the subthalamic nucleus in Parkinson's disease. *Brain*, Vol.123 (Pt 10), pp. 2091-2108

Sanchez-Ramos J.R., Ortoll R. & Paulson G.W. (1996).Visual hallucinations associated with Parkinson's disease. *Archives of Neurology*, Vol.53, pp. 1265-1268

Schroeder U., Kuehler A., Haslinger B. et al. (2002). Subthalamic nucleus stimulation affects striato-anterior cingulate cortex circuit in a response conflict task: a PET study. *Brain*, Vol.125, pp. 1995–2004

Schroeder U., Kuehler A., Lange K.W. et al. (2003). Subthalamic nucleus stimulation affects a frontotemporal network: a PET study. *Annals of Neurology*, Vol.54, pp. 445–50

Schupbach W. M., Chastan N., Welter M.L. et al. (2005). Stimulation of the subthalamic nucleus in Parkinson's disease: a 5 year follow up. *Journal of Neurology, Neurosurgery and Psychiatry*, Vol. 76, No.12, pp. 1640-1644

Schupbach W. M., Maltete D., Houeto J.L. et al. (2007). Neurosurgery at an earlier stage of Parkinson disease: a randomized, controlled trial. *Neurology*, Vol.68, No.4, pp. 267-271

Sensi M., Eleopra R., Cavallo M.A. et al. (2004). Explosive-aggressive behavior related to bilateral subthalamic stimulation. *Parkinsonism and Related Disorders*, Vol.10, No.4, pp. 247-51

Smeding H.M., Goudriaan A.E., Foncke E.M. et al. (2007). Pathological gambling after bilateral subthalamic nucleus stimulation in Parkinson disease. *Journal of Neurology, Neurosurgery and Psychiatry*, Vol. 78, No.5, pp. 517-9

Smeding H.M., Speelman J.D., Huizenga H.M. et al. (2011). Predictors of cognitive and psychosocial outcome after STN DBS in Parkinson's Disease. *Journal of Neurology, Neurosurgery and Psychiatry*, Vol. 82, No.7, pp. 754-60

Soulas T., Gurruchaga J.M., Palfi S. et al. (2008). Attempted and completed suicides after subthalamic nucleus stimulation for Parkinson's disease. *Journal of Neurology, Neurosurgery and Psychiatry*, Vol.79, No.8, pp. 952-954

Takeshita S., Kurisu K., Trop L. et al. (2005). Effect of subthalamic stimulation on mood state in Parkinson's disease: evaluation of previous facts and problems. *Neurosurgery Review, Vol.* 28, No.3, pp. 179-186

Taylor A.E., Saint-Cyr J.A. & Lang A.E. (1986). Frontal lobe dysfunction in Parkinson's disease: evidence for a "frontal lobe syndrome". *Brain and cognition*, Vol. 13, pp. 211-232

Tan S.K.H., Hartung H., Sharp T., et al. (2011). Serotonin-dependent depression in Parkinson's disease: a role for the subthalamic nucleus? *Neuropharmacology* Vol. 61, No. 3, pp. 387-399

Temel Y., Kessels A., Tan S. et al. (2006). Behavioural changes after bilateral subthalamic stimulation in advanced Parkinson disease: a systematic review. *Parkinsonism Related Disorders* Vol.12, No.5, pp. 265-272

Temel Y., Boothman L.J., Blokland A. et al. (2007). Inhibition of 5-HT neuron activity and induction of depressive-like behavior by high-frequency stimulation of the subthalamic nucleus. *Proceedings of the National Academy of Sciences of the United States of America* , Vol.23, No.104(43), pp. 17087-92

Thobois S., Ardouin C., Lhommée E. et al. (2010). Non-motor dopamine withdrawal syndrome after surgery for Parkinson's disease: predictors and underlying mesolimbic denervation. *Brain*, Vol. 133(Pt 4), pp. 1111-1127

Torack R.M. & Morris J.C. (1988). The association of ventral tegmental area histopathology with adult dementia. *Archives of Neurology*, Vol.45, No.5, pp. 497-501

Trepanier L.L., Kumar R., Lozano A.M. et al. (2000). Neuropsychological outcome of GPi pallidotomy and GPi or STN deep brain stimulation in Parkinson's disease. *Brain and Cognition, Vol.*42, pp. 324-47

Tröster A.I., Fields J.A., Wilkinson S.B. et al. (1997). Unilateral pallidal stimulation for Parkinson's disease: neurobehavioral functioning before and 3 months after electrode implantation. *Neurology*, Vol.49, No.4, pp. 1078-83

Tröster AI, Woods SP & Fields JA (2003). Verbal fluency declines after pallidotomy: an interaction between task and lesion laterality. *Applied Neuropsychology*, Vol.10, pp. 69-75.

Ulla M., Thobois S., Lemaire J.J. et al. (2006). Manic behaviour induced by deep brain stimulation in Parkinson's disease: evidence of substantia nigra implication? *Journal of Neurology, Neurosurgery and Psychiatry*, Vol.77, No.12, pp. 1363-1366

Ulla M., Thobois S. & Llorca P.M. (2011). Contact dependent reproducible hypomania induced by deep brain stimulation in Parkinson's disease: clinical, anatomical and functional imaging study. *Journal of Neurology, Neurosurgery and Psychiatry*, Vol.82, No.6, pp. 607-14

Umemura A., Oka Y., Okita K. et al. (2011). Subthalamic nucleus stimulation for Parkinson disease with severe medication-induced hallucinations or delusions. *Journal of Neurosurgery*, Vol.114, No.6, pp. 1701-5

Valldeoriola F., Nobbe F.A. & Tolosa E. (1997). Treatment of behavioral disturbances in Parkinson's disease. *Journal of Neural Trasmission (Suppl.)* Vol. 51, pp. 175-204

Van Wouwe N.C., Ridderinkhof K.R., van den Wildenberg W.P. et al. (2011). Deep brain stimulation of the subthalamic nucleus improves reward-based decision-learning in Parkinson's disease. *Frontiers in Human Neurosciences*, Vol.4, pp.5-30

Vingerhoets G., van der Linden C. & Lannoo E. (1999). Cognitive outcome after unilateral pallidal stimulation in Parkinson's disease. *Journal of Neurology, Neurosurgery and Psychiatry*, Vol.66, No.3, pp. 297-304

Visser-Vandewalle V., van der Linden C., Temel Y. et al. (2005). Long-term effects of bilateral subthalamic nucleus stimulation in advanced Parkinson disease: a four year follow-up study. *Parkinsonism Related Disorders*, Vol. 11, No.3, pp. 157-165

Volkmann J., Allert N., Voges J. et al. (2004). Long-term results of bilateral pallidal stimulation in Parkinson's disease. *Annals of Neurology*, Vol. 55, No.6, pp. 871-5

Voon V., Krack P., Lang A.E. et al. (2008). A multicentre study on suicide outcomes following subthalamic stimulation for Parkinson's disease. *Brain*, Vol. 131(Pt 10), pp. 2720-2728.

York M.K., Dulay M., Macias A. et al. (2008). Cognitive declines following bilateral subthalamic nucleus deep brain stimulation for the treatment of Parkinson's disease. *Journal of Neurology, Neurosurgery and Psychiatry*. Vol. 79, No.7, pp. 789-95

Yoshida F., Miyagi J., Kishimoto J. et al. (2009). Subthalamic nucleus stimulation does not cause deterioration of preexisting hallucinations in Parkinson's disease patients. *Stereotactic Functional Neurosurgery*, Vol. 87, No.1, pp. 45-49

Weintraub D., Koester J., Potenza M.N. et al. (2010). Impulse control disorders in Parkinson disease: a cross-sectional study of 3090 patients. *Archives of Neurology.*, Vol.67, No.5, pp. 589-95

Williams A.E., Arzola G.M. & Strutt A.M. (2011). Cognitive outcome and reliable change indices two years following bilateral subthalamic nucleus deep brain stimulation. *Parkinsonism Related Disorders*. 2011, Vol.17, No.5, pp. 321-7

Witt K., Pulkowski U., Herzog J. et al. (2004). Deep brain stimulation of the subthalamic nucleus improves cognitive flexibility but impairs response inhibition in Parkinson disease. *Archives of Neurology*, Vol.61, pp. 697–700

Witt K., Daniels C., Reiff J. et al. (2008). Neuropsychological and psychiatric changes after deep brain stimulation for Parkinson's disease: a randomised, multicentre study. *Lancet Neurology*, Vol. 7, No.7, pp. 605-614

Witjas T., Baunez C., Henry J.M. et al. (2005). Addiction in Parkinson's disease: impact of subthalamic nucleus deep brain stimulation. *Movement Disorders*, Vol. 20, No.8, pp. 1052-1055

Xuereb J.H., Tomlison B.E., Irving D. et al. (1990). Cortical and subcortical pathology in Parkinson's disease: relationship to parkinsonian dementia. In: *Parkinson's disease: anatomy, pathology and therapy*, M.B. Streiffler M.B., Korczyn A.D., Melamed E., Youdim M.B. 35-40, Advances in Neurology, vol. 53. , Raven Press Ltd , New York

Zahodne L.B., Susatia F., Bowers D. et al. (2011) Binge eating in Parkinson's disease: prevalence, correlates and the contribution of deep brain stimulation. *Journal of Neuropsychiatry and Clinical Neurosciences*, Vol. 23, No.1, pp. 56-62

Zangaglia R., Pacchetti C., Pasotti C. et al. (2009) Deep brain stimulation and cognitive functions in Parkinson's disease: A three-year controlled study. *Movement Disorders*, Vol. 15, No.24(11), pp. 1621-8

Zibetti M., Pesare M., Cinquepalmi A. et al. (2009). Neuro-psychiatric therapy during chronic subthalamic stimulation in Parkinson's disease. *Parkinsonism Related Disorders*, Vol. 15, No.2, pp. 128-133

Section 3

Advanced Techniques in Neurosurgery

6

Robotic Catheter Operating Systems for Endovascular Neurosurgery

Shuxiang Guo, Jian Guo, Nan Xiao and Takashi Tamiya
Kagawa University
Japan

1. Introduction

With the quickening pace of modern life, the brain diseases of people are increasing, such as cerebral aneurysm and infarction and so on. The traditional surgery spends patients a lot of operation time and has long recovery time, the burden on patients is heavy. Intracavity intervention is expected to become increasingly popular in the medical practice, both for diagnosis and for surgery. A lot of diagnosis and medical surgery with an endoscope or a catheter are performed for minimally invasive surgery recently. There are a lot of advantages as earliness etc. However, it requires a lot of skills for the operation so that this may do the operation in the inside of the body that cannot be watched directly.

Such surgery presents many challenges:

1. Doctors must be very well trained and possess the skills and experience to insert catheters. Intravascular neurosurgery is much more difficult than traditional surgery and there are few skilled doctors who can perform this type of operation. To keep pace with the growing number of patients, a mechanism is required to allow the training of sufficient numbers of doctors.
2. During the operation, doctors check the position of the catheter tip using the X-ray camera. Although they wear protective suits, it is very difficult to shield the doctor's hands and face from the effects of the X-ray radiation, which may result in radiation-related illness after long periods of exposure. The skilled surgeons operate the catheter using their hands directly, the conceptional scheme is shown in Fig.1.
3. In intravascular neurosurgery, catheters are inserted into the patient's blood vessels, which in the brain are very sensitive. When operating in this area, extreme care is required to avoid damaging the fragile vessels. An experienced neurosurgeon can achieve an accuracy of about 2 mm. However, as the contact force between the blood vessel and the catheter cannot be judged accurately by the doctor, so how to measure the contact force and feedback to the surgeon become significant.
4. Sometimes doctors cannot be physically present to operate on patients. Therefore, Internet-based master-slave systems are required for such cases so that the operation can be proceeded.

According to the above background, we developed two kinds of novel robotic catheter operating systems with danger avoiding method respectively, using the developed danger avoiding method it can not only help surgeons to know the situation inside blood vessel, but also can support surgeon to improve safety of operating process during intravascular neurosurgery. They can also provide the force feedback to the surgeon. We did experiment "In Vitro" to prove the feasibility of the developed first robotic catheter system, and we did evaluation for the second developed robotic catheter system.

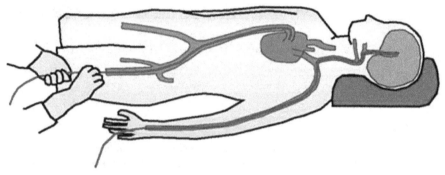

Fig. 1. Operating catheter with surgeon's hand

2. Relative products and researches on robotic catheter systems

In the past, there were a lot of researches and products on robotic catheter system. One of the more popular products is ANGIO Mentor endovascular surgical training simulator [OKB Medical], which is shown in Fig.2, it is a virtual reality (VR) simulator system, which can be used to train unskilled surgeon to do the operation of intravascular neurosurgery. However, it lacks of force feedback to the surgeons.

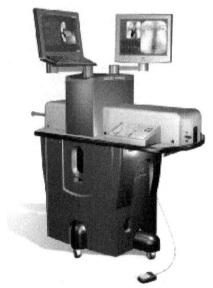

Fig. 2. ANGIO Mentor endovascular surgical training simulator

Another popular product is the Sensei robotic catheter system offered by Hansen Medical [Hansen Medical], which is shown in Fig.3, it can provide more precise manipulation with less radiation exposure to the doctor, however, force detection at the distal tip is very hard.

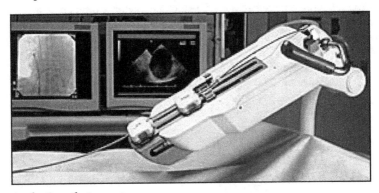

Fig. 3. Sensei robotic catheter system

Active catheter systems with SMA and ICPF as actuators were developed [S.Guo1996], new catheter driving method using linear stepping mechanism for intravascular neurosurgery has been developed [F.Arai2002], remote catheter navigation systems have been reported by [G. Srimathveeravalli2010], [Yogesh Thakur2009], [T.Goto2009], [E. Marcelli2008], and so on. Furthermore, the master-slave catheter systems were also developed [Y.Fu2011]. Although these products and catheter system have been developed, most concern is still the safety of the system. Force information of the catheter during the operation is very important to insure the safety of the surgery. A potential problem with a remote catheter control system is the lack of mechanical feedback. However, detection of the force on catheters is very hard to solve in these systems. In order to solve the problems, in this paper we proposed two kinds of novel robotic catheter systems with force feedback and monitoring image. They can provide the force feedback to the surgeon in real time.

3. Design of intelligent force sensors system

During the operation of intravascular neurosurgery, it is significant to obtain the contact force information between catheter and blood vessel [Christopher R. Wagner2002]. How to get it? And how to transmit it to the surgeon? In order to detect the contact force information between catheter and blood vessel, we developed an intelligent force sensors system for robotic catheter systems. By using the developed force sensors system, we can obtain the contact force information and feedback it to the surgeon. If there are no force sensors on the catheter, it is easy to damage the blood vessel during operating, because the blood vessel is fragile. The Fig.4 shows the comparison of safety between without force sensors on catheter and with force sensors on catheter.

3.1 Development of micro force sensors

The state-of-the-art in force and tactile sensing for minimally invasive surgery (MIS) has been reported [P. Puangmali2008], it presents the significance of the tactile sensor in MIS. Some tactile force sensors have been reported for the application of intravascular neurosurgery [R. Sedaghati2005], [K. Takashima2005, 2007], a micro force sensor on the catheter tip has been used in previous studies [Jan Peirs2004], and so on. However, these could only detect the contact force between the catheter head and the blood vessels, the frictional force and contact force between the side of catheter and blood vessel wall were not been paid attention. In order to solve above existed problems, in this paper, novel micro tactile force sensors were developed to measure the frictional force and contact force between blood vessel and the side of the catheter. The prototype of the developed tactile force sensors are shown in Fig.5, which are made of pressure sensitive rubber, their sizes are 4.0×4.0×0.5 mm and are fixed on the side wall of catheter by a linking shape.

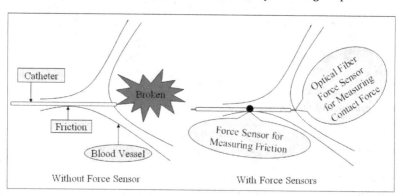

Fig. 4. Comparison of safety between two situations (Without force sensors and with force sensors)

A micro optical force sensor was used to measure front end force of the catheter, meanwhile, the optical fibre force sensor was served as guide wire to lead the catheter for inserting and rotating. The FOP-M optical fibre force sensor of FISO Technologies Inc. was used this time in our research.

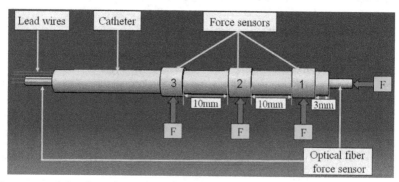

Fig. 5. Prototype of developed force sensors system

3.2 Calibration for the developed tactile force sensors

The calibration of the developed tactile force sensors was done, the calibration system is shown in Fig. 6, which consists of an electronic balance, a serial electric circuit, an oscilloscope, a power supply and a force load, we adjust the force load to different scale, the electronic balance will become different value, the tactile force sensor is loaded different value with force load, the tactile sensor output is different, the calibration results are shown in Fig.7, they indicated the relationship between load force and sensor output, based on the calibration results, we can obtain the concrete force output information of tactile sensors during the operation.

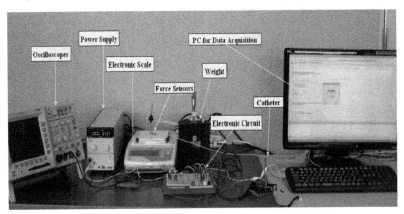

Fig. 6. Calibration system for the developed force sensors

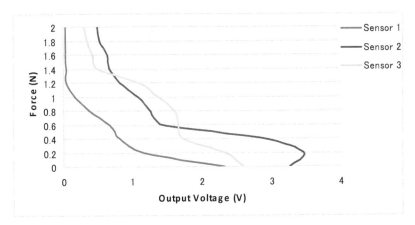

Fig. 7. Calibration results for the developed force sensors

3.3 Curve fitting equation for the calibration results

Based on the calibration results, we establish an equation between sensor outputs and load force using Matlab curve fitting tool, it is shown in equation (1), and we can also obtain the coefficient of equation for sensor1, sensor2 and sensor3, it is shown in table 1. Matlab curve fitting results for tactile force sensors are shown in Fig.8.

According to this equation, we can get the detail force output value of developed tactile force sensors if the tactile force sensors touch the blood vessel wall. Through the concrete force output value, surgeon can monitor the situation which catheter contact with the blood vessel sidewall.

$$f = c_{i3}v^3 + c_{i2}v^2 + c_{i1}v + c_{i0} \quad (i = 1,2,3) \tag{1}$$

Coefficient	Sensor 1	Sensor 2	Sensor 3
Ci3	-0.4762	-0.1874	-0.03155
Ci2	2.075	1.368	0.2049
Ci1	-2.97	-3.406	-1.15
Cio	1.668	3.25	2.145

Table 1. Coefficient of proposed cubic equation

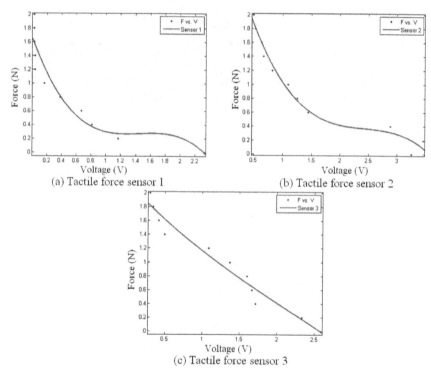

(a) Tactile force sensor 1
(b) Tactile force sensor 2
(c) Tactile force sensor 3

Fig. 8. Matlab curve fitting results for tactile force sensors

3.4 Force monitoring system

A force display method for a catheter operating system has been developed [J.Guo et al 2010], this method distinguished the force from developed force sensors to three ranges, safe range, danger warning range and dangerous range, however, this force display method did not show the detail force information at any moment, so surgeons could not know the concrete force information at any time, therefore, we improved the force information monitoring method so that surgeon can know the detail information at any moment during the operation, Fig.9 shows the force information monitoring system on the master side.

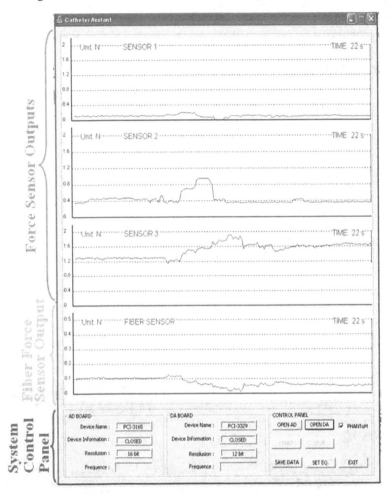

Fig. 9. Force information monitoring system

The novel force information monitoring method consists of two parts, sensor outputs part and system control panel part, which can monitor the changed force that catheter contact with blood vessel wall real time during the operation, in the sensor outputs part, it is divided four areas, three developed tactile force sensor outputs display areas and an optical fibre force sensor output display area. We can control the master-slave system in the system control panel part. Three tactile force sensors were used to measure the side force of catheter, and an optical force sensor was used to detect the front end force of catheter, if the force sensors touch the blood vessel, the output of force sensors will be shown in the force monitoring system real time, at the same time, the force feedback signals will be sent to the Phantom Omni, further more, The situation of operation can be monitored using web camera. In the master side, surgeons can not only monitor the force variation real time, but also they can feel the force feedback through Phantom Omni, when the contacted force is exceeded safe value, the Phantom Omni will be locked, so the developed system can automatically avoid the danger, and it can help surgeon improve the safety effectively during the operation.

4. Robotic catheter operating systems

Our research group developed two kinds of robot-assisted catheter system in the past, one kind is with haptic device called Phantom Omni as master manipulator, the other kind is with the master manipulator which can imitate surgeon's operating skill to insert and rotate catheter, we will introduce them as follows:

4.1 The first developed robotic catheter operating system

The first developed robotic catheter operating system is shown in Fig.10, at master side, the surgeon sees the monitoring image and operates the Phantom Omni, at the same time, the controlling instructions were transmitted to the slave side, after receiving the controlling instructions from master side, the slave manipulator drives the catheter to insert and rotate. Bu using the web camera to monitor the situation of operation, and by using force sensors to measure the contact force between catheter and blood vessel, the monitoring image and feedback force were transmitted to the surgeon in real time, based on the feedback force and monitoring image, the surgeon decides whether to insert the catheter or not. The flow chart of control signals is shown in Fig.11.

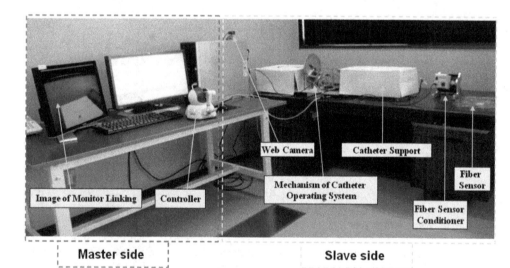

Fig. 10. The first developed master-slave robotic catheter system

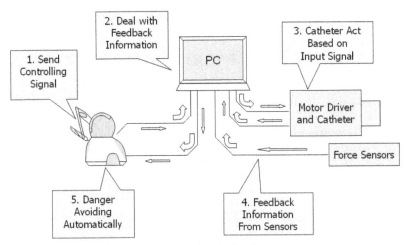

Fig. 11. Flow chart of control signals for first kind of catheter system

4.1.1 Master manipulator

The master manipulator is shown in Fig.12, called Phantom Omni, it is a haptic device, in this research, it was used to control the action of catheter, including inserting motion and rotating motion, we also use it to realize force feedback to avoid danger during operation of intravascular neurosurgery, when the force sensors contacted with blood vessel, the force feedback will be transmitted to the surgeon's hand in real time, if the contact forces exceeded warning force value, the Phantom Omni will be locked, so the developed catheter operating system can avoid the danger automatically, and it can help surgeon improve the safety effectively during the operation.

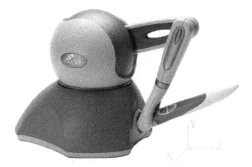

Fig. 12. Coordinate system of Phantom Omni

In order to realize the force feedback using Phantom Omni, the mechanical model of Phantom Omni was established, it is as follows:

The Phantom Omni output force $\bar{F}$ is:

$$\bar{F} = xi + yj + zk \tag{2}$$

Z direction is the inserting direction.

X direction is the rotating direction.

$$x \cdot z \equiv 0 \qquad (3)$$

f_1, f_2, f_3 is the forces that were measured by the developed force sensors.

f_4 is the force that was measured by the optical fibre force sensor.

When catheter is inserted, the Phantom Omni output force is as follows:

$$\vec{F} = 0 \cdot i + 0 \cdot j + A_i k$$

$$A_i = \{ \begin{array}{ll} 0 & (f_4 < C_0) \\ k \cdot f_4 & (f_4 > C_0) \end{array} \quad (k < 0) \qquad (4)$$

When catheter is rotated, the Phantom Omni output force is as follows:

$$\vec{F} = A_r \cdot i + 0 \cdot j + 0 \cdot k$$

$$f_{max} = \max(f_1, f_2, f_3) \qquad (5)$$

$$A_r = \{ \begin{array}{ll} 0 & (f_{max} < C_1) \\ k \cdot f_{max} & (f_{max} > C_1) \end{array} \quad (k < 0)$$

.

Based on the mechanical model of Phantom Omni, the force feedback output from Phantom Omni can be obtained, the value of the Phantom Omni force feedback is the force that surgeon feels. So the haptic force feedback can be realized by Phantom Omni and force sensors.

4.1.2 Slave manipulator

The conception of slave manipulator is shown in Fig.13, it can realize two motions for catheter, one is axial motion (moving forward and back-ward), and the other is radial motion (rotation). The catheter mostly moves forward and backward. When meeting the branch of blood vessel or moving difficulty, the catheter must rotate in order to enter the branch of blood vessel or get across block.

The mechanism of slave manipulator is shown in Fig.14, we make use of stepping motors as the actuators for driving the catheter. They can control the catheter moving to different directions. Considering the weight of mechanism, the whole mechanism is made of aluminium. The base of mechanism is made of stainless steel in order to increase the stabilization.

4.1.3 Experimental set up

We carried out the remote operating simulation experiment "in Vitro" using developed master-slave system in the simulator of blood vessel with an aneurysm, the simulator of blood vessel is made by silicon glass tube, which is shown in Fig.15. It is considered whose conditions are similar to those of a blood vessel of human brain.

Through the remote operating simulation experiment, we can measure the contact force between blood vessel wall and the catheter by developed micro tactile force sensors and optical fibre force sensor. Using the developed force monitoring system, we can obtain the outputs from micro tactile force sensors and optical fibre force sensor.

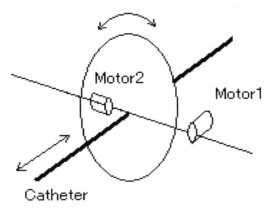

Fig. 13. Conception of slave manipulator

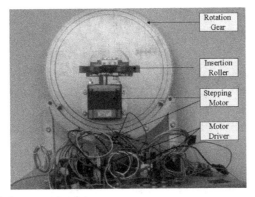

Fig. 14. Mechanism of slave manipulator

The experimental results are shown in Fig.16, Fig.17 and Fig.18. The output of developed tactile sensors are shown in Fig.16, the output of optical fibre force sensor is shown in Fig.17, making use of the mechanical model of Phantom omni, we can get the force feedback output of Phantom Omni, which is shown in Fig.18. From the graph we can know the relationship between operating time and force feedback from force sensors, and also we can know the force value when force sensors contact the simulator of blood vessel. It can also prove that the Phantom Omni is sensitive, and also it can avoid the danger automatically. The experimental results indicated that the developed novel type catheter operating system with force information monitoring method works properly, it can measure the contact force between catheter and blood vessel, also we can monitor the situation of simulation experiment using web camera, this catheter operating system can be controlled by teleoperation, and it can effectively improve the operability of aneurysm with force feedback for intravascular neurosurgery.

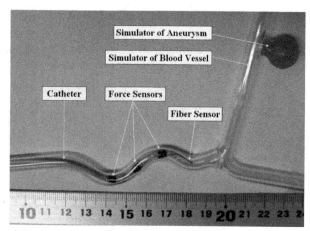

Fig. 15. Experimental set up

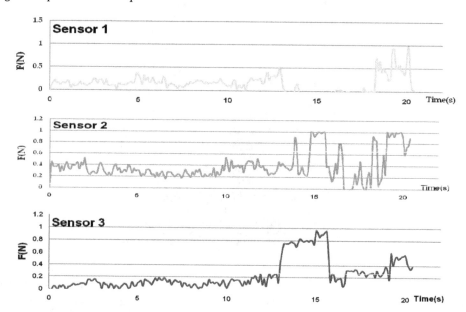

Fig. 16. Force outputs of developed tactile force sensors

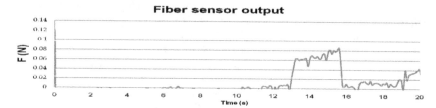

Fig. 17. Force output of optical fibre force sensor

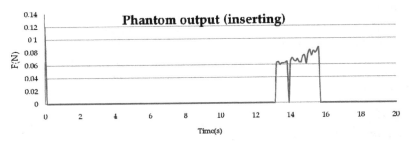

Fig. 18. Force feedback output of Phantom Omni

4.2 The second developed robotic catheter operating system

Because the Phantom manipulator can not imitate the operating skill of surgeon, we developed the other kind of robotic catheter system to simulate surgeon's operating skill for doing the operation of intravascular neurosurgery. Conceptual scheme of the second kind of robotic catheter system is shown in Fig.19. The flow chart of control signals for second kind of catheter system is shown in Fig.20.

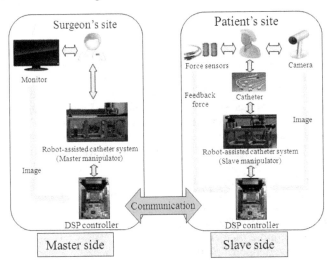

Fig. 19. Conceptual scheme of the second kind of robotic catheter system

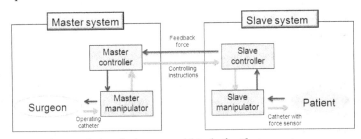

Fig. 20. Flow chart of control signals for second kind of catheter system

4.2.1 Master manipulator

On the master side, the slide platform is fixed on the supporting frame (Fig.21). The master system devices, including a left handle with one switch, a right handle, step motor, load cell, and maxon motor, are on the slide platform. The step motor is used to drive the slide platform forward and backward, the load cell is used to measure the operating force of surgeon's hand.

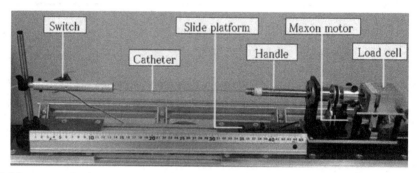

Fig. 21. Master manipulator

4.2.2 Slave manipulator

The slave side consists of a catheter clamping device, two DC motors, a slide platform, step motor, maxon motor, load cell, torque sensor, and support frame. The slave side mechanism shown in Fig.22 is similar to the master side; a slide platform is fixed on the supporting frame. The devices of the slave system are on the slide platform. The step motor is used to the drive slide platform forward and backward and the maxon motor is used to rotate the catheter. The two DC motors are used to control the catheter clamp. The load cell is used to measure the force between the catheter and blood vessel wall and the torque sensor and maxon motor are used to measure the force of catheter rotation. The measured force information is transmitted to the surgeon's hand, so that the surgeon can feel the feedback information from the slave side. A switch on the left handle on the master side controls the catheter clamp. When the surgeon wants to insert or rotate the catheter, clamp 2 is raised and clamp 1 clamps the catheter. The catheter navigator moves forward with the catheter for insertion or rotation. Clamp 2 then clamps the catheter; clamp 1 is raised and the catheter navigator moves backward. Repeating these actions, the actions of the slave side follow the commands of the master side in real time. If the catheter contacts the blood vessel wall, the force information is detected and transmitted to the surgeon's hand.

4.2.3 Mechanism control

In order to ensure the consistency and stability of the robotic catheter system, for both the rotating and inserting motions, a proportional-integral-derivative (PID) control method was developed for the robotic catheter operating system. A numerical simulation indicated that the response of the system was good using the PID control method. Furthermore, we did a simulation experiment using the robotic catheter system with the PID control strategy. The experimental results show that the response and consistency were good, enabling a surgeon to perform intravascular neurosurgery.

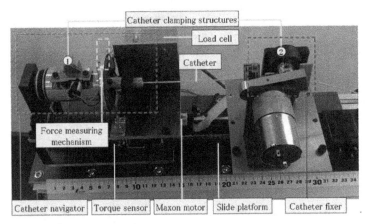

Fig. 22. Slave manipulator

4.2.3.1 Control strategy for inserting motion

We used the PID algorithm to assure accurate inserting motion, while reducing the hysteresis in real time. The following dynamic equation represents the control in the inserting direction:

$$F(t) = m\,\ddot{x}(t) + c\,\dot{x}(t) + kx(t) \tag{6}$$

Where F(t) is the force applied by the operator, $x(t)$, $\dot{x}(t)$, and $\ddot{x}(t)$ are the displacement, velocity, and acceleration of the operator's hand, respectively, m is the quality of the robotic catheter operating system (on the slide platform on the master side), c is the viscous damping coefficient, and k is the stiffness.

When the operator operates the right handle on the master side, the load cell measures the force. Using a dynamic equation based on the relationship between the operating force and resistance, the PID control strategy is used to adjust the consistency of the operating force in order to avoid overshoot. Fig.23 outlines the control of the inserting motion. The parameters of the operating system are as follows:

$$m = 2kg, c = 0.02N\,/\,(m\,/\,s), k = 10N\,/\,m$$

As on the master side, based on the input and output of the step motor, we used the same PID control strategy on the slave side to control the consistency and response of the slave mechanism during insertion.

4.2.3.2 Control strategy for rotating motion

Equation (7) represents the torque balance for the rotating motion on the master side, where m is the quality of the catheter operating system (on the slide platform on the master side), c is the viscous damping coefficient, $m = 2kg, c = 0.02N\,/\,(m\,/\,s)$, θ is the angle of rotation, u(t) is the variation in the torque, which is the torque of the maxon motor, $\dot{\theta}$ is the angular velocity, and $\ddot{\theta}$ is the angular acceleration. The control of rotation is shown in Fig.24.

$$m\ddot{\theta} + c\dot{\theta} = u(t) \tag{7}$$

As on the master side, based on the input and output of the maxon motor, we used the same PID control strategy on the slave side to ensure the consistency and response of the slave mechanism for rotation.

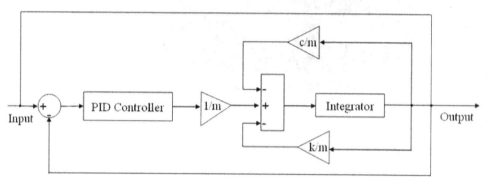

Fig. 23. The control of the insertion

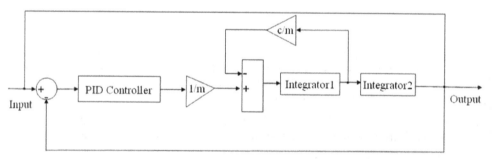

Fig. 24. The control of rotation

4.3 Catheter inserting experiment in vitro

In order to validate the robotic catheter operating system, we performed a simulation experiment to evaluate the characteristics of the master-slave robotic catheter operating system using an endovascular evaluator (EVE) (Fig. 25), which consisted of a fluid control unit and blood pressure monitoring instrument. The bending angles and radii of the tubes in the EVE are close to those of human arteries. The tubes were made of silicon rubber. The elasticity of the tubes was similar to that of a blood vessel wall. In order to keep the blood pressure of the EVE close to the blood pressure of a human, the fluid control unit was used to adjust the blood pressure, which was monitored with the blood pressure monitoring instrument. The operator operates the right handle on the master side to insert and rotate the catheter, which is inserted into the EVE from the femoral artery, controlling the speed and position of the catheter. The simulation experiment is shown in Fig. 26.

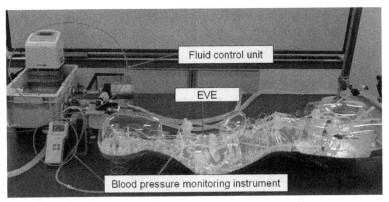

Fig. 25. The fluid control unit and blood pressure monitoring instrument of EVE

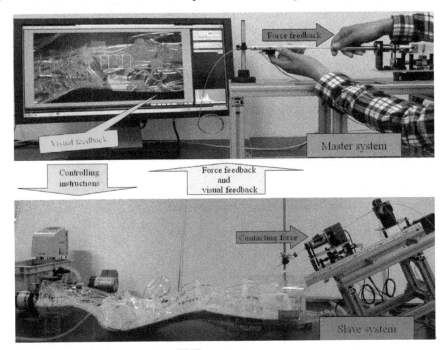

Fig. 26. Simulation experiment using EVE

4.3.1 Experimental results

We evaluated the robotic catheter system in a simulation experiment. Fig. 27 shows the results for the inserting motion, where the x-axis is the time axis and the y-axis is the displacement of the right handle on the master side (blue curve) and the catheter on the slave side (red curve). An upward slope is forward movement and a downward slope is backward movement. Fig. 28 shows the evaluation of rotation, where the x-axis is the time axis and the y-axis is the rotation of the right handle on the master side (blue curve) and the catheter on the slave side (red curve). From Figs. 27 and 28, the motions of the slave side follow the operating motions of the master side coincide very well in real time.

The measured insertion force is shown in Fig. 29, and this is also the feedback force transmitted to the operator's hand. The force sensors measure the contact force between the catheter and blood vessel wall. The fibre force sensor measures the force between the tip of the catheter and the blood vessel wall, the output of the fibre force sensor is shown in Fig. 30.

The experimental results indicate that our robotic catheter system can be used to perform VIS, without risk. The insertion force of the catheter is measured and fed back to the operator's hand, as is the contact force measured by the force sensors.

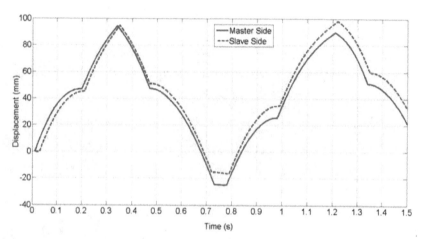

Fig. 27. Evaluated results for catheter insertion

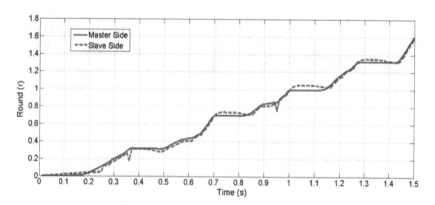

Fig. 28. Evaluated results for catheter rotation

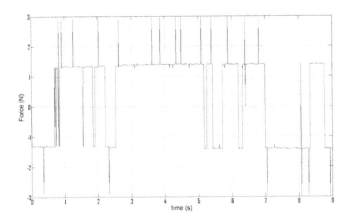

Fig. 29. The feedback force from the slave side

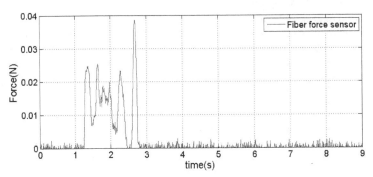

Fig. 30. The output of the fibre force sensor

4.3.2 Discussion

A simulation experiment was performed to validate our robotic catheter system. In order to enhance the stability and consistency of the robotic catheter system, we used a PID control strategy. The experimental results indicate that the response and consistency of the system were good, enabling a surgeon to perform VIS. It can also be used to train surgeons to insert and rotate a catheter for VIS smoothly. Nevertheless, due to the accuracy of the measuring device, the robotic catheter system is not ideal. In the future, we will improve the system. In addition, in the simulation experiment we used distilled water with a lubricant to simulate blood. Since the viscosity of distilled water differs from that of blood, the experimental results will differ slightly from an actual operation. We plan to improve the system by conducting animal experiments.

5. Conclusions

This paper presents two kinds of robotic catheter operating systems, they can assist surgeons to do the operation of intravascular neurosurgery, in addition, we designed a intelligent force sensors system to detect the contact force information between catheter and blood vessel, and also, we have done the simulation experiment "In Vitro" by using first developed robotic catheter system, the experimental results indicated that the first developed robotic catheter system work well, it can avoid danger automatically. We evaluated the second robotic catheter operating system via experiment in vitro by using EVE model, the evaluated results present that the second robotic catheter system can imitate the surgeon's operating skill to insert and rotate catheter, it is suitable for training unskilled surgeons to do the operation of intravascular neurosurgery. In the future, we will do some experiment in vivo by using the robotic catheter system.

6. Acknowledgment

This research is supported by Kagawa University Characteristic Prior Research fund 2011.

7. References

C. Preusche, T. Ortmaier, G. Hirzinger.(2002), Teleoperation concepts in minimal invasive surgery. Control Engineering Practice, 2002; 10:1245-1250.

C.R. Wagner, Nicholas Stylopoulos, Robert D. Howe(2002), The role of force feedback in surgery: analysis of blunt dissection, the Tenth Symposium on Haptic Interfaces for Virtual Environment and Teleoperator System, 2002.

E. Marcelli, L. Cercenelli, G. Plicchi.(2008), A novel telerobotic system to remotely navigate standard electrophysiology catheters, Computer in Cardiology 2008; 35:137-140.

F. Arai, R. Fujimura, T. Fukuda, M. Negoro.(2002), New catheter driving method using linear stepping mechanism for intravascular neurosurgery. Proceedings of the 2002 IEEE International Conference on Robotic & Automation, 2002; pp. 2944-2949.

G. Srimathveeravalli, T. Kesavadas, X. Li.(2010), Design and fabrication of a robot mechanism for remote steering and positioning of interventional devices, International Journal of Medical Robotics and Computer Assisted Surgery 2010; 6:160-170.

Hansen Medical, http://www.hansenmedical.com/sensei

J. Wang and S. Guo, H. Kondo, J. Guo and T. Tamiya.(2008), A Novel Catheter Operating System with Force Feedback for Medical Applications, International Journal of Information Acquisition, Vol.5, No.1, pp.83-91, 2008.

J. Peirs, Joeri Clijnen, Dominiek Reynaerts, Hendrik Van Brussel, Paul Herijgers, Brecht Corteville, et. al.(2004), A micro optical force sensor for force feedback during minimally invasive robotic surgery, Sensors and Actuators, Vol.115, No.2-3, pp.447-455, 2004.

J. Guo, N. Xiao, S. Guo.(2010), A force display method for a novel catheter operating system, Proceedings of the 2010 IEEE International Conference on Information and Automation, 2010; pp. 782-786.

J. Guo, N. Xiao, S. Guo, T. Tamiya.(2010), Development of a force information monitoring method for a novel catheter operating system, Information: An International Interdisciplinary Journal, 2010; 1(6):1999- 2009.

K. Takashima, K. Yoshinaka, T. Okazaki, K. Ikeuchi.(2005), An endoscopic tactile sensor for low invasive surgery. Sensors and Actuators A 2005; 119:372-383.

K. Takashima, R. Shimomura, T. Kitou, H. Terada, K. Yoshinaka, K. Ikeuchi.(2007), Contact and friction between catheter and blood vessel. Tribology International 2007; 40:319-328.

OKB Medical, http://www.okbmedical.com/angio

P. Puangmali, K. Althoefer, L.D. Seneviratne, D. Murphy, P. Dasgupta.(2008), State-of-the-art in force and tactile sensing for minimally invasive surgery. IEEE Sensors Journal, 2008; 8(4):371-381.

P. Polygerinos, T. Schaeffter, L. Seneviratne, K. Althoefer.(2009), Measuring tip and side forces of a novel catheter prototype: a feasibility study, Proceedings of the 2009 International Conference on Intelligent Robots and System, 2009; pp. 966-971.

Q. Pan, S. Guo, T. Okada.(2011), A novel hybrid wireless microrobot, International Journal of Mechatronics and Automation, 2011; 1(1):60-69.

R. Sedaghati, J. Dargahi, H. Singh.(2005), Design and modeling of an endoscopic piezoelectric tactile sensor, International Journal of Solids and Structures, Vol.42, No.21-22, pp.5872–5886, 2005.

S. Abdulla, P. Wen.(2011), Robust internal model control for depth of anaesthesia, International Journal of Mechatronics and Automation, 2011; 1(1):1-8.

S. Guo, Hidekazu Kondo, Jian Wang, Jian Guo, Takashi Tamiya.(2007) A New Catheter Operationg System for Medical Applications. Proceedings of the 2007 IEEE/ICME International Conference on Complex Medical Engineering, pp. 82-87, 2007.

S. Guo, Tatsuya Nakamtra, Toshio Fukuda, Keisuke Oguro, and Makoto Negoro. (1996), Micro Active Catheter Using ICPF Actuator Characteristic Evaluation, Proceedings of IEEE the 22nd Annual International Conf. on Industrial Electronics, Control, and Instrumentation, pp.1312-1317, 1996.

T. Fukuda, S. Guo, K. Kosuge, F. Arai, M. Negoro, and K. Nakabayash. (1994), Micro Active Catheter System with Multi Degree of Freedom, Proceedings of 1994 IEEE International Conference on Robotic and Automation, Vol.3, pp. 2290-2295, 1994.

T. Goto, T. Miyahara, K. Toyoda, J. Okamoto, Y. Kakizawa, J. Koyama, M. G. Fujie, K. Hongo.(2009), Telesurgery of microscopic micromanipulator system "NeuRobot" in neurosurgery: Interhospital Preliminary Study, Journal of Brain Disease 2009; 1:45-53.

X. Wang, M. Meng.(2011), Perspective of active capsule endoscope: actuation and localization, International Journal of Mechatronics and Automation, 2011; 1(1):38-45.

Y. Fu, A. Gao, H. Liu, S. Guo.(2011), The master-slave catheterization system for positioning the steerable catheter, International Journal of Mechatronics and Automation, 2011; 1(3), in press.

Y.C. Wu, J.S. Chen.(2011), Toward the identification of EMG-signal and its bio-feedback application, International Journal of Mechatronics and Automation, 2011; 1(2):112-120.

Y. Thakur, Jeffrey S. Bax, David W. Holdsworth and Maria Drangova.(2009), Design and performance Evaluation of a remote catheter navigation system, IEEE Transactions on Biomedical Engineering, Vol.56, No.7, July 2009, pp:1901-1908.

7

The Role of Neural Stem Cells in Neurorestoration

E.O. Vik-Mo, A. Fayzullin, M.C. Moe, H. Olstorn and I.A. Langmoen
Vilhelm Magnus Laboratory,
Department of Neurosurgery and Institute of Surgical Research, Oslo University Hospital
Norway

1. Introduction

Many neurological diseases have a poor prognosis. Most neurological treatment is primarily based on minimizing secondary - or further damage – and to optimize the remaining neurological function. Even a highly successful treatment like deep brain stimulation for Parkinson's disease improves neurological function through conditional lesioning. Several neurodegenerative diseases have no established treatments[1].

The complex electrochemical, molecular and anatomical structure of the central nervous system is established during prenatal and early postnatal development. Thus, it was long considered impossible to heal or substitute destroyed nervous tissue. The adult human brain used to be viewed as static, as it was a common perception that no new neurons could be generated after birth. This has been referred to as the "no new neurons"-dogma[2], and it goes back to the early neuronanatomist and Nobel Prize laureate Santiago Ramon y Cajal, who stated that "nothing may regenerate in the brain or central nervous system, everything may die"[3]. This axiom was challenged in the 1960s, but the work by Joseph Altman and co-workers was met with skepticism and was generally not accepted by the scientific community[4, 5].

During the 1970`s and 80`s Fernando Nottebohm and his colleagues made some very important discoveries. They found that the vocal centers in the brain of male canaries increase in size prior to the breeding season when vocal activities escalate to play pivotal roles in mating. In a series of studies they found no proliferation in the vocal centers, but showed that cell divisions took place in the ventricular wall. The newborn neurons then migrated to the vocal centers where they were integrated in neuronal circuits[6].

Evidence for neurogenesis in the mammalian brain was first presented by Reynolds and Weiss in 1992. They isolated cells from the striatum of adult mice and induced proliferation by epidermal growth factor[7]. Subsequently subsets of the cells developed the morphology and antigenic properties of neurons and astrocytes. Some of the newly generated cells also expressed immunoreactivity for the neurotransmitters typically found in that area of the adult mouse brain. In 1998 Eriksson et al. identified cells with stem cell characteristics *in situ* in the brain of adult humans post mortem[37, 152].

Through a steadily improving knowledge, primarily over the last 20 years, we have found that the central nervous system harbors cells with the ability to divide, mature and restore function after damage. Through manipulation it is even possible to differentiate cells derived from other organs into functioning neural cells that could be used as treatments.

A new approach, based on regeneration of central nervous tissue, might allow for better treatments for several of these devastating diseases. Although awaited with great hope, the translation of this basic research into tested treatments for patients is still wanting.

2. Definition of neural stem cells

Stem cells (SC) can loosely be described as cells that (I) have capacity for self-renewal (symmetric division), and (II) can give rise to cells other than themselves through asymmetric cell division[8]. SCs give rise to more differentiated progeny; **progenitor cells**. These cells have a more restricted ability for proliferation and differentiation.

The development from a multipotent stem cell to a variety of differentiated progeny has been most thoroughly examined in the hematopoietic system[9]. Here a detailed set of surface markers and transcription factors has been described to identify stem cells and different subsets of progenitor and differentiated cells[10]. Such a molecular phenotyping of the hierarchical organization allows for a detailed functional description, and to form hypothesis readily testable. However, even in this relatively well characterized cellular hierarchy controversies exist both on the stem cell nature and on the correct phenotype of such cells.

Cells with SC characteristics that can give rise to neural tissue or are derived from the central nervous system (CNS) are called neural stem cells (NSC). NSC can be derived from several sources. In principal such cells can be classified according to the sources of origin. Cells can be isolated from embryos, fetal, or the adult CNS. Neural stem cells are multipotent, giving rise to the three major cell types of the mammalian CNS: neurons, astrocytes and oligodendrocytes. Adult stem cells, also referred to as somatic stem cells, are undifferentiated cells found among mature and specialized cells in a tissue or organ, and reside in various tissues in the human body, including the central nervous system. It is the stem cells of the adult brain that drive adult neurogenesis.

The hierarchy of somatic stem cell differentiation in solid tissue is however much less clear[11, 12]. In addition, little is known about the differentiation pathways from such stem cells into the main groups of cells comprising brain stroma. Suggested progenitor cell phenotypes may differ between different parts of the brain[13, 14]. The fact that there exist thousands of different types of neurons in the CNS adds magnitudes of complexity. The impact of *in vitro* cultural artifacts confuses available data even further. Similar problems of stem- and progenitor-cell identification are present in several other organ systems where somatic stem cells have been described (breast, lung, prostate, skin, and gut). With such an uncharted landscape, defining a definitive SC population clearly poses a great problem.

Several approaches have been used to isolate and identify potential NSC. After the successful use of flow cytometry for identification of SC in the hematopoietic system, surface markers have been sought for NSC. The marker CD133 (also termed prominin-1 or AC133) was initially identified on a subset of human hematopoietic stem and progenitor cells [15]. Antibodies directed at this protein were shown to prospectively identify a population of progenitor cells isolated from fetal human brain tissue[16]. CD133 is also expressed by the slow-dividing fraction of human umbilical cord progenitor cells[17]. This marker has been identified in the subventricular zone (SVZ) and rostral migratory stream [18] and even cortex [19] in human post-mortem derived tissue. Conflicting data exist however[20, 21], where a group identified CD133 positive cells in cells derived from embryonic SC, ependymal cells and brain tumor cells – but not in neurogenic cells derived from the adult human subventricular zone. This discrepancy may be due to technical issues, but could also be related to the plasticity of these cells in vitro as CD133 levels seems to be affected by bioenergetic stress[22-24]. Due to the discrepancy between studies, other adult human neural stem cell (ahNSC) or precursor markers have been suggested (SSEA1, CXCR4, A2B5, peanut-agglutinin ++)[21, 25]. These are less explored, but all seem to struggle with the level of variability and heterogeneity.

SCs are more robust than differentiated cells. The fact that NSC can be isolated from human brain >48 hrs post mortem exemplifies this fact[26]. Another well known example is the regrowth of hair lost during chemotherapy treatment. During chemotherapy patients loose hair one to three weeks after initiation of therapy. However, the SC of hair follicles survive, and usually hair grow back from three to six months after termination of therapy[27]. The molecular machinery behind increased DNA-repair mechanisms, free-radical scavengers systems and membrane pumps to expel toxic substances have been described in a range of cancers[28]. The presence of the same molecular machinery in a variety of malignancies implies that such mechanisms are based on activation of intrinsic cellular properties and signaling events. The molecular machinery allowing protection of somatic stem cells could be used to prospectively identify and enrich for such cells. The efflux of toxic substances by ABC (ATP Binding Cassette Transporter) membrane pumps was used to identify a population of cells with high efflux of the DNA-binding dye Hoechst 33342 with stem cell properties in murine hematopoietic system [29]. This functional phenotype was identified in fractions of cells isolated from developing mouse brain [30] and brain tumor cell lines [31]. Similarly, the ability to metabolize aldehydes has been used to identify stem cells in developing and adult murine brain[32]. Whether this approach will overcome the problems described above for surface markers is still unknown.

A third approach is to enrich for stem cells using culturing conditions selectively allowing for these cells to proliferate. This has been shown to effectively allow NSC proliferation in a range of species (murine[33], canine[34], porcine[35], monkey[36] and human[37]). Similarly, non-adherent, serum-poor culturing conditions have been shown to be applicable for SC in colon[38, 39], breast[40, 41], prostate[42,43], heart[44], skin[45, 46], pancreas[47, 48], and liver[49]. Under these conditions SC can proliferate extensively, while cells lacking this ability are eliminated. The demonstration of extensive self-renewal and generation of differentiated progeny by a large number of groups have shown this to be a robust method of isolating SC.

3. Neurogenesis and biology of endogenous NSCs

3.1 Neurogenesis and neurogenic regions

Stem cells differentiating into neurons (neurogenesis) have been identified in both the dentate gyrus of the hippocampus and in the walls of the lateral ventricles in the subventricular zone (SVZ) and the rostral migratory stream (RMS) - the main pathway by which newly born neurons from SVZ reach the olfactory bulb. Cells in both neurgenic niches seem to translate through similar cellular development, but the anatomical organization is quite different.

In the dentate gyrus cells migrate only a few micrometers, from the subgranular zone to the granule cell layer. Cells develop from a precursor cell type in which mitotic events are found. Most of the newly formed cells are eliminated, and only few cells are able to establish axons, dendrites and functional synapses (postmitotic maturation phase). During the late survival phase characteristic electrophysiological patterns develop, receiving glutamatergic input from the entorhinal cortex and sending out axons to the hippocampal CA3 region. After a maturation period of several weeks the newly developed neurons establish characteristics identical to the other preexisting neurons[2].

The SVZ, in the walls of the lateral ventricles, contains the largest concentration of dividing cells in the adult mammalian brain[4, 50]. In the human brain there seems to be far more proliferating cells in the SVZ compared to the hippocampus[51, 52]. The cellular composition and organization of this region differs somewhat amongst species[53, 54]. In mammals the SVZ contains three cell populations important for stem cell proliferation. The proper stem cell population is maintained through slowly dividing astrocyte-like neural stem cells known as type B cells. These cells give rise to actively proliferating type C cells, which in turn give rise to immature neuroblasts, called type A cells. These neuroblasts, not yet neuronally committed, migrate to the olfactory bulb via chain migration by cell-cell contacts. Neuroblast chains are ensheathed by the processes of type B cells. In the anterior and dorsal SVZ, these chains condense to form the RMS [55-57]. After reaching the olfactory bulb cells migrate radially along blood vessel, and differentiate into interneurons incorporated into the functional circuitry of olfactory bulb and forebrain[50, 57].

In the adult brain, rodent and human studies reveal that neurogenesis continues in the SVZ throughout adult life[4, 56, 58-60]. The SVZ-RMS structure of the human brain contains 10^5 dividing cells, a number that is high compared with the rodent[51, 61]. As age increases in rodents, the number of neurogenic cells decreases[62, 63]. Early data based on magnetic resonance spectroscopy suggests that this may also be the case in humans[64].

Under normal circumstances the function of the SVZ is to produce neuroblasts for the RMS[51, 53, 56]. More recent experiments have demonstrated that the progenitors of the SVZ are capable of producing oligodendrocytes in addition to olfactory interneurons[65]. After experimental injury in animal models of Huntigton disease and stroke, the SVZ not only supplies the RMS with neuroblasts but SVZ progenitor cells also migrate toward the site of injury and cell death[66, 67]. Thus, the proliferation and migration from the SVZ responds to injury, suggesting a more important role for this region in neurorestoration.

3.2 Regulatory signaling of the NSC pool

The proliferation and differentiation of the NSC pool is highly regulated. The microenvironment maintaining this function is called the stem cell niche. This is a combination of signaling through extracellular matrix (ECM), cell-cell contacts, secreted substances, innervation and physical factors.

The niche is embedded in extensions of the vascular basal lamina that extends around NSCs and progenitors[68]. These laminin and collagen I-rich ECM structures can be observed under the electron microscope and have been named fractones. These structures has been suggested to bind secreted growth factors, like Fiborblast growth factor (FGF), regulating concentrations and signaling strength of secreted factors[69, 70], tenascin-C[70-72], osteopentin[73], chondroitin/dermatan sulfate proteoglycans[74, 75].

Ependymal cells, lining the ventricles, exert a supporting/ regulatory function in the niche, since they can modulate the transport of ions and other factors from the cerebrospinal fluid (CSF)[76]. They secrete neurogenic factors like pigment epithelium-derived factor (PEDF)[77] and the pro-neurogenic bone morphogenic protein (BMP) signaling substances[78, 79]. These cells also form gap junctions with SVZ astrocytes[80], allowing controlled transfer of substances from the CSF to the niche. NSC adapt close contacts to blood vessels both in the subgranular zone and the SVZ[69, 81]. This connection is suggested to be central in neurogenesis[82]. This could be through cell-cell-contact mediated signaling or through secreted factors like PEDF, leukemia-inhibitory factor (LIF) and brain-derived neurotrophic factor (BDNF) [83].

Several studies have shown effect on SVZ progenitor proliferation through infusion of growth factors into the ventricles. FGF, epidermal growth factor (EGF) and transforming growth factor alpha (TGFalpha)[62, 84, 85] have no identified source within the niche, but may originate from the choroid plexus and transported through CSF. Platelet derived growth factor (PDGF), PEDF and Vascular endothelial growth factor (VEGF) derived from endothelial cells regulate NSC and progenitor proliferation[77, 86-88], and PDGF also have effects on the differentiational balance between neurons and oligodendrocytes[86]. Several other secreted factors contributes to this orchestra of regulation like LIF[87, 89], BDNF[90, 91] and BMPs[78, 92].

Of special interest are the three stem cell related signaling pathways; Hedgehog-, Wnt- and Notch- pathways. Sonic hedgehog (Shh) is a morphogen known to regulate neurogenesis and gliogenesis during development. This signaling increase precursor and NSC proliferation both in the hippocampus and the SVZ[94-96] and Shh is essential for their maintenance[97]. Genetic manipulation by knocking-down the Shh signaling results in depletion of SVZ neurogenesis, while increased signaling leads to upregulation of proliferation[98]. Wnt-pathway signaling is orchestrated through a number of secreted Wnt ligands and a range of Frizzled receptors, and their interaction mediates the possibility for fine tuning of a proliferation-differentiation signal[99-102]. The combination of FGF and b-catenin signaling might be a requisite for neuronal differentiation[103]. Notch signaling is based on binding of ligands and receptors that are membrane bound, and thus acts through cell-cell interaction. This signaling is essential for niche maintenance, and again regulates both the size of the NSC pool and differentiation[104, 105], and differences in Notch signaling distinguish NSC from progenitors[106].

The convergence of synaptic input by classical neurotransmitters like γ-amino-butyric acid (GABA) and serotonin (5-HT) modulates the NSC niche. GABA is the principle inhibitory neurotransmitter in the adult CNS but has an excitatory action in the SVZ and the subgranular zone of the hippocampus[107, 108]. This effect is similar to its effect during brain development [109]. Isolated rat neuroblasts also express the GABA-A receptor. GABA has been found to decrease neuroblast migration[110] and to cause cell cycle exit[111], suggesting that the number of dividing neuroblasts could be regulated by a feedback loop between NSCs and neuroblasts[112]. Major focus has been put on the serotonergic systems effect on the niche due to its importance in psychiatric diseases [113]. Early studies depleting serotonin (5-HT) in prenatal stages showed a reduction in cell proliferation in both neurogenic niches[114]. The effects of 5-HT are mediated on receptor level on NSC population might, however, differ in the SVZ and the subgranular layer[115, 116].

In Huntington's disease (HD) the SVZ increases in size, and has increased number of progenitor cells, while the mature cells present are altered. In Parkinson disease, on the other hand, the number of proliferating progenitors is almost halved compared to the normal situation[66, 67, 117-119]. This is believed to be related to the loss of dopamine stimulation of NSC proliferation.

Gas composition also affects NSC regulation. Processes of nitrergic neurons intercalate with neuroblasts in the SVZ [120]. Inhibitors of Nitirc oxide (NO) signaling affects cell proliferation and NO synthase deficient mice also exhibit higher levels of proliferation in the SVZ[120-122]. Oxygen tension highly affects the potency and proliferative potential of NSC[123, 124], and can switch the neurogenesis from differentiation of GABA-positive to glutamate positive neurons[125].

3.3 Cancer stem cells and their relation to NSC

The phenotype of neural stem cells is mirrored in several aspects of malignant tumor biology[126-128]. Several of the intrinsic molecular pathways and extracellular signaling systems identified in regulation of NSC have also been identified in cancer cells. Such cells, termed cancer stem cells (CSC) have been suggested to be essential in tumor growth and therapy resistance. Since NSC harbor the molecular machinery to respond to signals of proliferation and defense mechanisms to extrude toxic substances[129, 130], it has been suggested that NSC are the cell of origin for brain neoplasms[131]. By using conditionally targeted gene knock down of the tumor suppressor p53 in neural progenitor cells (Nestin +) and astrocytes (GFAP+), it has been demonstrated that both populations of cells can give rise to tumors[132, 133]. The induction of tumors however seem to be at lesser threshold by RAS and AKT transformation in Nestin+ cells, suggesting greater risk of tumor development from less differentiated cells. Similarly, different cell populations of NSCs, neural progenitor cells (NPCs) and more differentiated cells can all be candidates for malignant transformation[131]. In two subgroups of medulloblastomas different cells of origin and different molecular pathways seem to be important in tumorigenesis. Midline medulloblastomas present in the brain stem seem to develop from dorsal brainstem progenitors and be dependent on the Wnt- pathway. More laterally situated, cerebellar tumors seem to develop from granule neuron progenitors and be stimulated through SHH-pathway signaling[134].

The NSC pool and niche is highly controlled through a range of factors, underscoring the biological importance of these cell populations. Manipulating the signaling pathways for NSC homeostasis could thus be potential therapeutic intervention in brain tumors. Conversely, it is apparent that molecular signals or drugs that induce NSC proliferation could potentially be tumorigenic.

4. Challenges for the generation of NSCs

Several stem cell types have neural capabilities: 1. pluripotent self-renewing embryonic stem cells, 2. multipotent stem cells with broad potential and self-renewing capacity from embryonic, fetal or adult brain, 3. neural progenitors with limited potential and self-renewal capacity from adult brain or spinal cord, 4. committed neural progenitors (neuronal and glial) from brain subregions [135].

Embryonic stem cells (ESCs) have an almost unlimited capacity to self-renew. On the other hand, ESCs also have a considerable teratogenic potential after implantation into host tissue, and it is not yet clear how long chromosomal stability can be maintained[136]. In addition, immense ethical concerns exist regarding the use of human ESCs as well as government restrictions that continue to limit clinical applications [137].

Human fetal mesencephalic NSCs fulfill some important requirements for the use in cell replacement strategies. They can be generate high yields of functional neurons from a small starting population, representing on-demand availability of cells without major logistical problems and the possibility to standardize the cell source in a clinical setting. In contrast to ES cells, tumorigenicity seems to be a minor problem with fetal NSCs. These cells are less flexible with regards to multiplication and differentiation, but there is increasing evidence that it is more beneficial to use cells that are already committed to becoming a particular cell type[138].

More recently, induced pluripotent stem cells (iPS) were generated, and such cells offer another source of autologous neural stem cells[137]. It has been known that differentiated cells can be reprogrammed to an embryonic-like state by nuclear transfer to oocytes, fusion with ES cells or molecular reprogramming of somatic cells into induced pluripotent stem cells using genetic factors[138]. Most of the current reprogramming methods are using expression of putative oncogenes by retroviral vectors. The factors used are involved in carcinogenesis, posing a risk for clinical translation. Important questions regarding safety and genetic stability must be solved before iPS can be used in clinical trials[139].

Brain-derived ahNSC are very attractive because of the clear logistical benefits if the therapeutic stem cells can be derived from a patient's own body. Technical obstacles (obtaining fetal and embryonic tissue, immune graft rejection in hetero- and xenotransplantation, potential tumor formation after grafting of induced pluripotent cells) as well as ethical issues (in contrast to embryonic, fetal, hetero- or xenotransplantations of cells) can be avoided. Despite this, there are limited data concerning the application of adult human-derived neural stem cells in clinical trials and very limited number of experimental data[140].

Adult human neural stem cells can be isolated from a range of sources. Cells derived from the two neurogenic regions of the brain have been the most thoroughly examined, but cells with neurogenic potential in vitro can be derived from subcortical white matter[141], spinal cord[142], filum terminale[143, 144] and hypothalamus[145]. Also cells derived from the olfactory mucosa, found in the nasal cavity, contain ahNSC[146]. Several of these regions allow for harvesting of autologous NSC with minimal risk and morbidity for the patient[143, 146, 147].

Multipotent adult stem cells have also significant advantages with regard to autologous transplantation approaches without immunological graft rejection. Hematopoietic stem cells

(HSCs) and mesenchymal stem cells (MSCs) are valuable sources for cell transplantation and cell therapy. Although recent *in vitro* as well as *in vivo* studies suggested that multipotent adult stem cells, or their pro-neurally converted derivatives, could display protective or regenerative effects in experimental models of CNS diseases[138], more experimental data to translate the application of this type of cells to clinical trial is needed[137].

The discovery of multipotent stem and progenitor cells in the adult human brain has opened the possibility of treating central nervous system disorders through replacement of the injured tissue by transplanted cells or by stimulating recruitment of endogenous repair mechanisms. We have previously shown that in principle adult human neural progenitor cells (ahNPCs) could be transplanted to ischemically damaged brain for in vivo maturation into neurons[93,148]. The latter can be achieved both by infusion of growth factors or by transplanting progenitors delivering neurogenic factors to the injured brain. .

To obtain such a goal, one must have culturing protocols with the ability to obtain enough cells resulting in a clinically significant effect in one or more patients. In addition, the cells must survive long enough for quality testing and possible genetic manipulation before transplantation. One of the main obstacles when culturing ahNPCs has been that the cells seem to stop proliferating after a limited number of passages and also lose their ability for proper differentiation with repetitive passages[151]

The problem may however not apply to all ahNSC, as olfactory mucosa derived SC show higher propencity for proliferation and have been shown to be effective in an animal model of PD[195]. Also, it has been reported that ahNPCs can be propagated *in vitro* for as long as 20 months (12 to 15 passages) and have shown differentiation into cells expressing neuronal and astrocytic markers[149]. Together with a publication by Walton et al.[150], this article provides further evidence that the limitations upon continued propagation of ahNPCs previously reported by others may be surmounted.

Finally, when an adequate number of cells have been produced in vitro, the cells must be documented to have the appropriate ability to differentiate into mature neurons with the ability to produce synapses and generate functional action potentials. While we have documented this in cells cultivated short term in vitro[151-153], similar data on long term cultivated cells are lacking. We are looking forward to future experiments we hope will evaluate the ability of these long-term propagated progenitors for normal functional differentiation in vitro and in vivo.

5. NSC treatment strategies

Concerning the techniques of NSC application, regardless of the cell source, there are several treatment strategies that are explored in restorative approach.

5.1 Stimulation of endogenous NSC

It is evident that the adult brain contains a pool of NSC that have the ability to proliferate and that can respond to extrinsic signals[154, 155].

Recent data suggests that NSCs and NPCs can migrate from their site of birth to other parts of the brain and contribute to the replacement of specific cell types lost due to injury or disease[156-158]. In animal stroke models striatal neurons can be derived from endogenous NSC and progenitors [157, 159-161]. Similarly, compensatory neurogenesis exists in Huntington's and Alzheimer's disease patients. Compensatory neocortical neuron production have been demonstrated after targeted ablation of both interneurons and corticospinal neurons[162-165]. This neurogenesis is, however, quite modest and not associated with clinically significant functional effects. This is probably due to the limited number of stem cells recruited and/or the unfavorable environment of the injured adult brain for supporting efficient production of new neurons and glia.

Thus, the current challenge is to understand how to modify the molecular basis of compensatory neurogenesis in order to overcome its limiting factors in the pathological and aged CNS, while supporting those that accentuate its' influence.

Several of the described factors that affects the NSC pool are potentially tumor inducing when administered systemically, thus a major obstacle in developing this type of therapy is how to deliver the factor- or rather- the sequence of factors needed at high temporal and anatomical precision. Animal models have primarily used intraventricular injections or viral delivery methods to achieve this. Intraventricular injection of TGFAlpha activates endogenous neurogenesis in the SVZ of Parkinson's disease (PD) model rats [166, 167]. Similarly, the injection of the Notch receptor ligand angiopoietin2 or Dll4 growth factors can induce widespread stimulation of endogenous neural precursors, and in a PD rodent model rescue injured dopamine neurons and stimulate improvement of motor function. Adenoviral co-delivery of BDNF and BMP signaling molecule Noggin induces striatal neuron replacement from endogenous precursors and delays motor impairment in a Huntington's disease model[168]. Intraventricluar injection of EGF and erythropoietin in combination can mobilize endogenous adult neural stem cells to promote cortical tissue re-growth and functional recovery after stroke[169]. Systemic erythropoietin is already in clinical use for the stimulation of erythropoiesis, thus allowing a rapid translation of this approach to clinical investigation. In a combination with the neurotrophic hormone β-human chorionic gonadotropin (hCG) this was found to be safe, and potentially beneficial in a phase II trial for the stimulation of neurogenesis after stroke[170].

5.2 Cell replacement by transplantation

As several obstacles remain regarding how to stimulate the correct cells with the correct sequence of stimulatory factors within the complex NSC niche, most therapeutic strategies are based on the transplantation of in vitro or ex vivo manipulated cells.

Most groups have favored the transplantation of immature cells. The idea is to let grafted cells differentiate under the influence of the host environment, integrate into the local neuronal network and thus become a functional unit of the brain or spinal cord. Immature cells are believed to be more robust than differentiated cells, and could contain the necessary plasticity to overcome pathological scar formation and inhibitory signals of relocation and differentiation. This approach is the most common in animal models of neurorestoration[2]. Also, the transplanted cells must have the ability to form the correct cells needed, and must stop proliferation when the proper cell types have been formed.

Better control of the developed progeny could be achieved by grafting of mature or at least partly differentiated cells. It is supposed that predifferentiation may help the processes of functional integration of transplanted cells. We have shown that in selective injury of hippocampal CA1 region by global ischemia both ahNSC and predifferentiated cells preferentially migrate into the damaged area[93,148]. The predifferentiated cells develop more markers of differentiated neurons at an earlier time point. Thus, ahNSC can be manipulated *in vitro* to yield a greater neuronal differentiation after transplantation. In approaches where potential tumor forming cells are used, a controlled differentiation could reduce the risk of adverse tumor formation[165]. Similar in-vitro predifferentiation has been tested for generation of dopaminergic neurons in PD[169]. Further modification of the transplanted cells could be genetically manipulated cells that secret anti-apoptotic or pro-differentiation signal or a combination of NSC and stromal cells.

5.3 Microenvironmental modification

A third approach facilitates the ability of transplanted cells to affect the environment which the cells are transplanted into. Autocrine and paracrine factors derived from NSC can modulate the niche and stem-, progenitor and differentiated cells after transplantation. In rats it has been found that secreted growth factors from transplanted NSCs stimulated proliferation of endogenous NSC[171], called "bystander effect". In several transplantation studies functional recovery is far greater than the number of identified transplanted cells would indicate. This has been suggested to be a result of synergistic effects of the NSC on the host microenvironment.

Furthermore, transplanted NSC can secrete factors not present in the host. Infantile neuronal ceroid lipofuscinosis is a fatal neurodegenerative disease caused by a deficiency in the lysosomal enzyme palmitoyl protein thioesterase-1 (PPT1). The lack of this enzyme leads to pathological lipofuscin-like material accumulating in cells, leading to progressive loss of vision, decreasing cognitive and motor skills, epileptic seizures and premature death. Normally functioning cells produce surplus of this enzyme, and some of this is secreted to the extracellular environment. This secreted enzyme can be absorbed by other cells, also cells not producing this enzyme on their own. This can be done in quantities high enough to stop lysosomal sequestering. In a mouse model lacking the gene for PPT1 transplanted NSC could reduce lipofuscine levels, provide neuroprotection and delay loss of motor function [172].

6. Towards using NSC to treat neurological disorders

Although NSC therapy have been suggested as a therapy for a range of neurological diseases, here we highlight the results for the most studied diseases; PD, stroke, and spinal cord injury.

6.1 Parkinson's disease

Over the past 30 years, neural transplantation has emerged as a possible therapy for PD. It was shown that grafted neural cells from different sources can survive for over 20 years and exert beneficial effects in PD patients[173]. Different types of cell have been tested both in experimental and clinical trial. Embryonic derived stem cells have been suggested the cell of choice, since they promise to be made in high quantities and to hold large amounts of the desired cell type [138]. Clinical testing of transplants to patients with PD of primary human embryonic dopaminergic neurons or tissue using double-blind, placebo-controlled protocols have shown positive results. The patients displayed impressive improvements of symptoms and restoration of dopaminergic neurotransmission, but also demonstrated several clinical limitations. Only subpopulations of patients showed significant clinical benefits. Moreover, a significant proportion of patients (with up to 56%) suffered from dyskinesias after a twelve-hour drug-free period[174-176].

Whether, these early results could be transferable to the use of ESC is uncertain. Also, the use of ÈSC harbors problems of controlling cell growth and differentiation, including brain tumor and teratoma formation[138, 177-179]. In contrast, there are no reports of tumor formation in fetal NSCs transplantations, what makes the usage of fetal tissue-specific be a safer way to establish a transplantation protocol in PD. Open-label clinical studies continued through the 1990s have shown that fetal ventral mesencephalic allografts could survive in patients with advanced PD, become functionally integrated, and produce sustained clinical benefits; however, it also soon became clear that transplants of this type produced very variable responses, with some patients showing only little improvement or transient benefits[173]. In patients receiving grafts post mortem studies have demonstrated that also transplanted cells display Lewy bodies, a sign of PD[180, 181].

Overall several issues hinders the further development of a cellular replacement approach for PD[176]. Ethical issues and technical problems (i.e. obtaining fetal and embryonic tissue, immune graft) are slowing down the clinical application in PD patients. New candidate for cell replacement are needed, but the role of other types of potential sources for transplantations - brain-derived adult neural stem cells, adult multipotent stem cells, induced pluripotent cells is still not clear. One case-report describes the effect of autologous transplantation of SVZ derived NSC[140]. Although effects on several clinical aspects were reported, these only lasted 36 months and weaned off after 4-5 years. Based on this result, a phase II study has been approved, but later put on hold due to demands put on cell production facilities (neurogeneration.com).

6.2 Stroke

Stroke is another severe pathology where significant loss of neural tissue is the major factor of the illness. No current therapies promote neuronal recovery following ischemic insults. As mentioned above, endogenous NSC proliferate as a response to both ischemic stroke and subarachnoid hemorrage[182, 183], and stimulation of this endogenous neurogenesis has been tried using a combination with of erythropoietin and hCG as mentioned above.

Based on work in animal models, transplantation of exogenous cells into the injured brain to replace the lost cells or support the remaining cells is one of promising direction[184]. There is a significant experimental background that supports the idea that the grafting of exogenous stem cells from multiple sources can generate neural cells that survive and form synaptic connections after transplantation in the stroke-injured brain[185]. The world's first fully regulated clinical trial of a neural stem cell therapy for disabled stroke patients - PISCES study (Pilot Investigation of Stem Cells in Stroke) – has been started in Scotland at the Institute of Neurological Sciences in 2011. Stem cell therapy (purified population of human neural stem cells, derived from human fetal brain tissue) is being administered to a total of 12 patients. The obtained data is planned to be announced in 2012.

6.3 Spinal cord injury

Cell replacement in spinal cord injury (SCI) is also a field of great interest for neurobiologist and clinicians. A large number of different cells including embryonic and adult stem cells have been transplanted into animal models of spinal cord injury, and in many cases these procedures have resulted in modest sensorimotor benefits[186]. Also a range of clinical experiments involving administration of stem cells for SCI patients have already taken place. Early studies in nine patients showed that unselected human fetal neural tissue transplanted to progressively developing posttraumatic syringomyelia could safely be used to obliterate the syrinx[187, 188]. No tumor developed, but the clinical effect of this obliteration was however limited.

A Portuguese study have reported using unselected olfactory mucosa transplanted into SCI damage site in twenty patients with complete medullary lesions[189, 190]. Treatment resulted in a filling at the transplant site. Urodynamic responses improved in five patients. Two of the patients regained voluntary control of anal sphincter. Eleven patients improved while one patient declined in ASIA impairment scale. The authors concluded that olfactory mucosa autografts are feasible, safe and possibly beneficial.

Geron Corporation (Menlo Park, CA, USA) was in 2009 given a US Food and Drug Administration (FDA) approval for the first test of human embryonic stem cell derived oligodendroglial cells in patients for SCI. Although high controversy existed regarding cell source, safety and patient selection, several patients were included into the study. After an early stop in the study because of worries regarding cyst development at injection sites in preclinical studies, recruitment started in 2010. In the first four patients included in the study, the treatment appeared safe. Sadly, the study was recently stopped due to financial reasons[191].

7. Future directions

Through the last two decades the presence and potential of NSC has become apparent. NSC are used to understand developments of pathology and new based treatments are explored in a range of neurological disease

Although we clearly are at a very early stage of translating the basic biological understanding of NSC into possible therapies, several phase I and II studies have been reported using cell based approaches to treat neurological conditions. However several obstacles affect the translation of promising preclinical studies. Laws, regulation and public understanding of this research are poorly developed. While ethical concerns have develop into regulations that forces restrictive use on a broad range of new technologies in some regions, lack of established safety and quality parameters have led to unsafe and dangerous trials other places[192]. It is a story as old as it is unfortunate, in which opportunistic individuals and companies may manipulate hype and hope for financial gain[193]. Already reports exist on patient developing tumors after ill-designed and unsafe treatment based on NSC[194]. Certainly, at this early stage NSC based therapies should be part of a well designed and publically reported clinical trial (http://www.isscr.org/clinical_trans/pdfs/ISSCRPatientHandbook.pdf).

8. References

[1] Gogel S, Gubernator M, Minger SL. Progress and prospects: stem cells and neurological diseases. Gene Ther 2011; 18(1):1-6.

[2] Kempermann G. Adult Neurogenesis. Stem Cells and Neuronal Development in Adult Brain. New York: Oxford University Press; 2006.

[3] Cajal R. Degeneration and Regeneration Nervous System. Oxford University Press; 1913.

[4] Altman J. Proliferation and migration of undifferentiated precursor cells in the rat during postnatal gliogenesis. Exp Neurol 1966; 16(3):263-278.

[5] Kornblum HI. Introduction to neural stem cells. Stroke 2007; 38(2 Suppl):810-816.

[6] Nottebohm F. Neuronal replacement in adulthood. Ann N Y Acad Sci 1985; 457:143-161.

[7] Reynolds BA, Weiss S. Generation of neurons and astrocytes from isolated cells of the adult mammalian central nervous system. Science 1992; 255(5052):1707-1710.

[8] Morrison SJ, Shah NM, Anderson DJ. Regulatory mechanisms in stem cell biology. Cell 1997; 88(3):287-298.

[9] Kawamoto H, Wada H, Katsura Y. A revised scheme for developmental pathways of hematopoietic cells: the myeloid-based model. Int Immunol 2010; 22(2):65-70.

[10] Giebel B, Punzel M. Lineage development of hematopoietic stem and progenitor cells. Biol Chem 2008; 389(7):813-824.

[11] Vickaryous MK, Hall BK. Human cell type diversity, evolution, development, and classification with special reference to cells derived from the neural crest. Biol Rev Camb Philos Soc 2006; 81(3):425-455.

[12] Croft AP, Przyborski SA. Formation of neurons by non-neural adult stem cells: potential mechanism implicates an artifact of growth in culture. Stem Cells 2006; 24(8):1841-1851.

[13] Alvarez-Buylla A, Kohwi M, Nguyen TM, Merkle FT. The heterogeneity of adult neural stem cells and the emerging complexity of their niche. Cold Spring Harb Symp Quant Biol 2008; 73:357-365.

[14] Stancik EK, Navarro-Quiroga I, Sellke R, Haydar TF. Heterogeneity in ventricular zone neural precursors contributes to neuronal fate diversity in the postnatal neocortex. J Neurosci 2010; 30(20):7028-7036.

[15] Yin AH, Miraglia S, Zanjani ED et al. AC133, a novel marker for human hematopoietic stem and progenitor cells. Blood 1997; 90(12):5002-5012.

[16] Uchida N, Buck DW, He D et al. Direct isolation of human central nervous system stem cells. Proc Natl Acad Sci U S A 2000; 97(26):14720-14725.

[17] Wagner W, Ansorge A, Wirkner U et al. Molecular evidence for stem cell function of the slow-dividing fraction among human hematopoietic progenitor cells by genome-wide analysis. Blood 2004; 104(3):675-686.

[18] Kam M, Curtis MA, McGlashan SR, Connor B, Nannmark U, Faull RL. The cellular composition and morphological organization of the rostral migratory stream in the adult human brain. J Chem Neuroanat 2009; 37(3):196-205.

[19] Schwartz PH, Bryant PJ, Fuja TJ, Su H, O'Dowd DK, Klassen H. Isolation and characterization of neural progenitor cells from post-mortem human cortex. J Neurosci Res 2003; 74(6):838-851.

[20] Pfenninger CV, Roschupkina T, Hertwig F et al. CD133 is not present on neurogenic astrocytes in the adult subventricular zone, but on embryonic neural stem cells, ependymal cells, and glioblastoma cells. Cancer Res 2007; 67(12):5727-5736.

[21] Sun Y, Kong W, Falk A et al. CD133 (Prominin) negative human neural stem cells are clonogenic and tripotent. PLoS One 2009; 4(5):e5498.

[22] Bar EE, Lin A, Mahairaki V, Matsui W, Eberhart CG. Hypoxia increases the expression of stem-cell markers and promotes clonogenicity in glioblastoma neurospheres. Am J Pathol 2010; 177(3):1491-1502.

[23] Griguer CE, Oliva CR, Gobin E et al. CD133 is a marker of bioenergetic stress in human glioma. PLoS One 2008; 3(11):e3655.

[24] Platet N, Liu SY, Atifi ME et al. Influence of oxygen tension on CD133 phenotype in human glioma cell cultures. Cancer Lett 2007; 258(2):286-290.

[25] Pfenninger CV, Roschupkina T, Hertwig F et al. CD133 is not present on neurogenic astrocytes in the adult subventricular zone, but on embryonic neural stem cells, ependymal cells, and glioblastoma cells. Cancer Res 2007; 67(12):5727-5736.

[26] Palmer TD, Schwartz PH, Taupin P, Kaspar B, Stein SA, Gage FH. Cell culture. Progenitor cells from human brain after death. Nature 2001; 411(6833):42-43.

[27] Trueb RM. Chemotherapy-induced alopecia. Curr Opin Support Palliat Care 2010; 4(4):281-284.

[28] Hanahan D, Weinberg RA. The hallmarks of cancer. Cell 2000; 100(1):57-70.

[29] Goodell MA, Brose K, Paradis G, Conner AS, Mulligan RC. Isolation and functional properties of murine hematopoietic stem cells that are replicating in vivo. J Exp Med 1996; 183(4):1797-1806.

[30] Murayama A, Matsuzaki Y, Kawaguchi A, Shimazaki T, Okano H. Flow cytometric analysis of neural stem cells in the developing and adult mouse brain. J Neurosci Res 2002; 69(6):837-847.

[31] Kondo T, Setoguchi T, Taga T. Persistence of a small subpopulation of cancer stem-like cells in the C6 glioma cell line. Proc Natl Acad Sci U S A 2004; 101(3):781-786.

[32] Corti S, Locatelli F, Papadimitriou D et al. Identification of a primitive brain-derived neural stem cell population based on aldehyde dehydrogenase activity. Stem Cells 2006; 24(4):975-985.

[33] Reynolds BA, Weiss S. Generation of neurons and astrocytes from isolated cells of the adult mammalian central nervous system. Science 1992; 255(5052):1707-1710.

[34] Milward EA, Lundberg CG, Ge B, Lipsitz D, Zhao M, Duncan ID. Isolation and transplantation of multipotential populations of epidermal growth factor-responsive, neural progenitor cells from the canine brain. J Neurosci Res 1997; 50(5):862-871.

[35] Dyce PW, Zhu H, Craig J, Li J. Stem cells with multilineage potential derived from porcine skin. Biochem Biophys Res Commun 2004; 316(3):651-658.

[36] Tonchev AB, Yamashima T, Sawamoto K, Okano H. Enhanced proliferation of progenitor cells in the subventricular zone and limited neuronal production in the striatum and neocortex of adult macaque monkeys after global cerebral ischemia. J Neurosci Res 2005; 81(6):776-788.

[37] Kukekov VG, Laywell ED, Suslov O et al. Multipotent stem/progenitor cells with similar properties arise from two neurogenic regions of adult human brain. Exp Neurol 1999; 156(2):333-344.

[38] Carpentino JE, Hynes MJ, Appelman HD et al. Aldehyde dehydrogenase-expressing colon stem cells contribute to tumorigenesis in the transition from colitis to cancer. Cancer Res 2009; 69(20):8208-8215.

[39] Ricci-Vitiani L, Lombardi DG, Pilozzi E et al. Identification and expansion of human colon-cancer-initiating cells. Nature 2007; 445(7123):111-115.

[40] Dontu G, Al-Hajj M, Abdallah WM, Clarke MF, Wicha MS. Stem cells in normal breast development and breast cancer. Cell Prolif 2003; 36 Suppl 1:59-72.

[41] Liu S, Dontu G, Mantle ID et al. Hedgehog signaling and Bmi-1 regulate self-renewal of normal and malignant human mammary stem cells. Cancer Res 2006; 66(12):6063-6071.

[42] Lawson DA, Witte ON. Stem cells in prostate cancer initiation and progression. J Clin Invest 2007; 117(8):2044-2050.

[43] Duhagon MA, Hurt EM, Sotelo-Silveira JR, Zhang X, Farrar WL. Genomic profiling of tumor initiating prostatospheres. BMC Genomics 2010; 11:324.

[44] Davis DR, Zhang Y, Smith RR et al. Validation of the cardiosphere method to culture cardiac progenitor cells from myocardial tissue. PLoS One 2009; 4(9):e7195.

[45] Le RH, Zuliani T, Wolowczuk I et al. Asymmetric distribution of epidermal growth factor receptor directs the fate of normal and cancer keratinocytes in vitro. Stem Cells Dev 2010; 19(2):209-220.

[46] Toma JG, Akhavan M, Fernandes KJ et al. Isolation of multipotent adult stem cells from the dermis of mammalian skin. Nat Cell Biol 2001; 3(9):778-784.

[47] Gaviraghi M, Tunici P, Valensin S et al. Pancreatic cancer spheres are more than just aggregates of stem marker-positive cells. Biosci Rep 2010; 31(1):45-55.

[48] Seaberg RM, Smukler SR, Kieffer TJ et al. Clonal identification of multipotent precursors from adult mouse pancreas that generate neural and pancreatic lineages. Nat Biotechnol 2004; 22(9):1115-1124.

[49] Uchida Y, Tanaka S, Aihara A et al. Analogy between sphere forming ability and stemness of human hepatoma cells. Oncol Rep 2010; 24(5):1147-1151.

[50] Lois C, varez-Buylla A. Proliferating subventricular zone cells in the adult mammalian forebrain can differentiate into neurons and glia. Proc Natl Acad Sci U S A 1993; 90(5):2074-2077.

[51] Curtis MA, Kam M, Nannmark U et al. Human neuroblasts migrate to the olfactory bulb via a lateral ventricular extension. Science 2007; 315(5816):1243-1249.

[52] Lucassen PJ, Meerlo P, Naylor AS et al. Regulation of adult neurogenesis by stress, sleep disruption, exercise and inflammation: Implications for depression and antidepressant action. Eur Neuropsychopharmacol 2010; 20(1):1-17.

[53] Doetsch F, Garcia-Verdugo JM, varez-Buylla A. Cellular composition and three-dimensional organization of the subventricular germinal zone in the adult mammalian brain. J Neurosci 1997; 17(13):5046-5061.

[54] Quinones-Hinojosa A, Sanai N, Soriano-Navarro M et al. Cellular composition and cytoarchitecture of the adult human subventricular zone: a niche of neural stem cells. J Comp Neurol 2006; 494(3):415-434.

[55] Lois C, varez-Buylla A. Long-distance neuronal migration in the adult mammalian brain. Science 1994; 264(5162):1145-1148.

[56] Lois C, Garcia-Verdugo JM, varez-Buylla A. Chain migration of neuronal precursors. Science 1996; 271(5251):978-981.

[57] Peretto P, Merighi A, Fasolo A, Bonfanti L. Glial tubes in the rostral migratory stream of the adult rat. Brain Res Bull 1997; 42(1):9-21.

[58] Benraiss A, Chmielnicki E, Lerner K, Roh D, Goldman SA. Adenoviral brain-derived neurotrophic factor induces both neostriatal and olfactory neuronal recruitment from endogenous progenitor cells in the adult forebrain. J Neurosci 2001; 21(17):6718-6731.

[59] Eriksson PS, Perfilieva E, Bjork-Eriksson T et al. Neurogenesis in the adult human hippocampus. Nat Med 1998; 4(11):1313-1317.

[60] Luskin MB, Boone MS. Rate and pattern of migration of lineally-related olfactory bulb interneurons generated postnatally in the subventricular zone of the rat. Chem Senses 1994; 19(6):695-714.

[61] Kam M, Curtis MA, McGlashan SR, Connor B, Nannmark U, Faull RL. The cellular composition and morphological organization of the rostral migratory stream in the adult human brain. J Chem Neuroanat 2009; 37(3):196-205.

[62] Kuhn HG, ckinson-Anson H, Gage FH. Neurogenesis in the dentate gyrus of the adult rat: age-related decrease of neuronal progenitor proliferation. J Neurosci 1996; 16(6):2027-2033.

[63] Luo J, Daniels SB, Lennington JB, Notti RQ, Conover JC. The aging neurogenic subventricular zone. Aging Cell 2006; 5(2):139-152.

[64] Manganas LN, Zhang X, Li Y et al. Magnetic resonance spectroscopy identifies neural progenitor cells in the live human brain. Science 2007; 318(5852):980-985.

[65] Menn B, Garcia-Verdugo JM, Yaschine C, Gonzalez-Perez O, Rowitch D, varez-Buylla A. Origin of oligodendrocytes in the subventricular zone of the adult brain. J Neurosci 2006; 26(30):7907-7918.

[66] Arvidsson A, Collin T, Kirik D, Kokaia Z, Lindvall O. Neuronal replacement from endogenous precursors in the adult brain after stroke. Nat Med 2002; 8(9):963-970.

[67] Tattersfield AS, Croon RJ, Liu YW, Kells AP, Faull RL, Connor B. Neurogenesis in the striatum of the quinolinic acid lesion model of Huntington's disease. Neuroscience 2004; 127(2):319-332.

[68] Mercier F, Kitasako JT, Hatton GI. Anatomy of the brain neurogenic zones revisited: fractones and the fibroblast/macrophage network. J Comp Neurol 2002; 451(2):170-188.

[69] Kerever A, Schnack J, Vellinga D et al. Novel extracellular matrix structures in the neural stem cell niche capture the neurogenic factor fibroblast growth factor 2 from the extracellular milieu. Stem Cells 2007; 25(9):2146-2157.

[70] Jaworski DM, Fager N. Regulation of tissue inhibitor of metalloproteinase-3 (Timp-3) mRNA expression during rat CNS development. J Neurosci Res 2000; 61(4):396-408.

[71] de CA, Lemasson M, Saghatelyan A, Sibbe M, Schachner M, Lledo PM. Delayed onset of odor detection in neonatal mice lacking tenascin-C. Mol Cell Neurosci 2006; 32(1-2):174-186.

[72] Kazanis I, Belhadi A, Faissner A, Ffrench-Constant C. The adult mouse subependymal zone regenerates efficiently in the absence of tenascin-C. J Neurosci 2007; 27(51):13991-13996.

[73] Sailor KA, Dhodda VK, Rao VL, Dempsey RJ. Osteopontin infusion into normal adult rat brain fails to increase cell proliferation in dentate gyrus and subventricular zone. Acta Neurochir Suppl 2003; 86:181-185.

[74] Akita K, von HA, Furukawa Y, Mikami T, Sugahara K, Faissner A. Expression of multiple chondroitin/dermatan sulfotransferases in the neurogenic regions of the embryonic and adult central nervous system implies that complex chondroitin sulfates have a role in neural stem cell maintenance. Stem Cells 2008; 26(3):798-809.

[75] von Holst A, Sirko S, Faissner A. The unique 473HD-Chondroitinsulfate epitope is expressed by radial glia and involved in neural precursor cell proliferation. J Neurosci 2006; 26(15):4082-4094.

[76] Bruni JE. Ependymal development, proliferation, and functions: a review. Microsc Res Tech 1998; 41(1):2-13.

[77] Ramirez-Castillejo C, Sanchez-Sanchez F, ndreu-Agullo C et al. Pigment epithelium-derived factor is a niche signal for neural stem cell renewal. Nat Neurosci 2006; 9(3):331-339.

[78] Lim DA, Tramontin AD, Trevejo JM, Herrera DG, Garcia-Verdugo JM, varez-Buylla A. Noggin antagonizes BMP signaling to create a niche for adult neurogenesis. Neuron 2000; 28(3):713-726.

[79] Peretto P, Dati C, De MS et al. Expression of the secreted factors noggin and bone morphogenetic proteins in the subependymal layer and olfactory bulb of the adult mouse brain. Neuroscience 2004; 128(4):685-696.

[80] Zahs KR. Heterotypic coupling between glial cells of the mammalian central nervous system. Glia 1998; 24(1):85-96.

[81] Palmer TD, Willhoite AR, Gage FH. Vascular niche for adult hippocampal neurogenesis. J Comp Neurol 2000; 425(4):479-494.

[82] Shen Q, Goderie SK, Jin L et al. Endothelial cells stimulate self-renewal and expand neurogenesis of neural stem cells. Science 2004; 304(5675):1338-1340.

[83] Riquelme PA, Drapeau E, Doetsch F. Brain micro-ecologies: neural stem cell niches in the adult mammalian brain. Philos Trans R Soc Lond B Biol Sci 2008; 363(1489):123-137.

[84] Craig CG, Tropepe V, Morshead CM, Reynolds BA, Weiss S, van der KD. In vivo growth factor expansion of endogenous subependymal neural precursor cell populations in the adult mouse brain. J Neurosci 1996; 16(8):2649-2658.

[85] Wagner JP, Black IB, Cicco-Bloom E. Stimulation of neonatal and adult brain neurogenesis by subcutaneous injection of basic fibroblast growth factor. J Neurosci 1999; 19(14):6006-6016.

[86] Jackson EL, Garcia-Verdugo JM, Gil-Perotin S et al. PDGFR alpha-positive B cells are neural stem cells in the adult SVZ that form glioma-like growths in response to increased PDGF signaling. Neuron 2006; 51(2):187-199.

[87] Jin K, Mao XO, Sun Y, Xie L, Greenberg DA. Stem cell factor stimulates neurogenesis in vitro and in vivo. J Clin Invest 2002; 110(3):311-319.

[88] Jin K, Zhu Y, Sun Y, Mao XO, Xie L, Greenberg DA. Vascular endothelial growth factor (VEGF) stimulates neurogenesis in vitro and in vivo. Proc Natl Acad Sci U S A 2002; 99(18):11946-11950.

[89] Mi H, Haeberle H, Barres BA. Induction of astrocyte differentiation by endothelial cells. J Neurosci 2001; 21(5):1538-1547.

[90] Leventhal C, Rafii S, Rafii D, Shahar A, Goldman SA. Endothelial trophic support of neuronal production and recruitment from the adult mammalian subependyma. Mol Cell Neurosci 1999; 13(6):450-464.

[91] Scharfman H, Goodman J, Macleod A, Phani S, Antonelli C, Croll S. Increased neurogenesis and the ectopic granule cells after intrahippocampal BDNF infusion in adult rats. Exp Neurol 2005; 192(2):348-356.

[92] Colak D, Mori T, Brill MS et al. Adult neurogenesis requires Smad4-mediated bone morphogenic protein signaling in stem cells. J Neurosci 2008; 28(2):434-446.

[93] Olstorn H, Varghese M, Murrell W, Moe MC, Langmoen IA. Predifferentiated brain-derived adult human progenitor cells migrate toward ischemia after transplantation to the adult rat brain. Neurosurgery 2011; 68(1):213-222.

[94] Ahn S, Joyner AL. In vivo analysis of quiescent adult neural stem cells responding to Sonic hedgehog. Nature 2005; 437(7060):894-897.

[95] Palma V, Lim DA, Dahmane N et al. Sonic hedgehog controls stem cell behavior in the postnatal and adult brain. Development 2005; 132(2):335-344.

[96] Wechsler-Reya RJ, Scott MP. Control of neuronal precursor proliferation in the cerebellum by Sonic Hedgehog. Neuron 1999; 22(1):103-114.

[97] Balordi F, Fishell G. Hedgehog signaling in the subventricular zone is required for both the maintenance of stem cells and the migration of newborn neurons. J Neurosci 2007; 27(22):5936-5947.

[98] Han YG, Spassky N, Romaguera-Ros M et al. Hedgehog signaling and primary cilia are required for the formation of adult neural stem cells. Nat Neurosci 2008; 11(3):277-284.

[99] Bonnert TP, Bilsland JG, Guest PC et al. Molecular characterization of adult mouse subventricular zone progenitor cells during the onset of differentiation. Eur J Neurosci 2006; 24(3):661-675.

[100] Garcia-Castro MI, Marcelle C, Bronner-Fraser M. Ectodermal Wnt function as a neural crest inducer. Science 2002; 297(5582):848-851.

[101] Lie DC, Colamarino SA, Song HJ et al. Wnt signalling regulates adult hippocampal neurogenesis. Nature 2005; 437(7063):1370-1375.

[102] Yu JM, Kim JH, Song GS, Jung JS. Increase in proliferation and differentiation of neural progenitor cells isolated from postnatal and adult mice brain by Wnt-3a and Wnt-5a. Mol Cell Biochem 2006; 288(1-2):17-28.

[103] Israsena N, Hu M, Fu W, Kan L, Kessler JA. The presence of FGF2 signaling determines whether beta-catenin exerts effects on proliferation or neuronal differentiation of neural stem cells. Dev Biol 2004; 268(1):220-231.

[104] Alexson TO, Hitoshi S, Coles BL, Bernstein A, van der KD. Notch signaling is required to maintain all neural stem cell populations--irrespective of spatial or temporal niche. Dev Neurosci 2006; 28(1-2):34-48.

[105] Chapouton P, Skupien P, Hesl B et al. Notch activity levels control the balance between quiescence and recruitment of adult neural stem cells. J Neurosci 2010; 30(23):7961-7974.

[106] Mizutani K, Yoon K, Dang L, Tokunaga A, Gaiano N. Differential Notch signalling distinguishes neural stem cells from intermediate progenitors. Nature 2007; 449(7160):351-355.

[107] Ge S, Pradhan DA, Ming GL, Song H. GABA sets the tempo for activity-dependent adult neurogenesis. Trends Neurosci 2007; 30(1):1-8.

[108] Wang DD, Krueger DD, Bordey A. GABA depolarizes neuronal progenitors of the postnatal subventricular zone via GABAA receptor activation. J Physiol 2003; 550(Pt 3):785-800.

[109] Owens DF, Liu X, Kriegstein AR. Changing properties of GABA(A) receptor-mediated signaling during early neocortical development. J Neurophysiol 1999; 82(2):570-583.

[110] Bolteus AJ, Bordey A. GABA release and uptake regulate neuronal precursor migration in the postnatal subventricular zone. J Neurosci 2004; 24(35):7623-7631.

[111] Overstreet WL, Bromberg DA, Bensen AL, Westbrook GL. GABAergic signaling to newborn neurons in dentate gyrus. J Neurophysiol 2005; 94(6):4528-4532.

[112] Liu X, Wang Q, Haydar TF, Bordey A. Nonsynaptic GABA signaling in postnatal subventricular zone controls proliferation of GFAP-expressing progenitors. Nat Neurosci 2005; 8(9):1179-1187.

[113] Santarelli L, Saxe M, Gross C et al. Requirement of hippocampal neurogenesis for the behavioral effects of antidepressants. Science 2003; 301(5634):805-809.

[114] Brezun JM, Daszuta A. Depletion in serotonin decreases neurogenesis in the dentate gyrus and the subventricular zone of adult rats. Neuroscience 1999; 89(4):999-1002.

[115] Banasr M, Hery M, Printemps R, Daszuta A. Serotonin-induced increases in adult cell proliferation and neurogenesis are mediated through different and common 5-HT receptor subtypes in the dentate gyrus and the subventricular zone. Neuropsychopharmacology 2004; 29(3):450-460.

[116] Radley JJ, Jacobs BL. 5-HT1A receptor antagonist administration decreases cell proliferation in the dentate gyrus. Brain Res 2002; 955(1-2):264-267.

[117] Curtis MA, Penney EB, Pearson AG et al. Increased cell proliferation and neurogenesis in the adult human Huntington's disease brain. Proc Natl Acad Sci U S A 2003; 100(15):9023-9027.

[118] Curtis MA, Waldvogel HJ, Synek B, Faull RL. A histochemical and immunohistochemical analysis of the subependymal layer in the normal and Huntington's disease brain. J Chem Neuroanat 2005; 30(1):55-66.

[119] Curtis MA, Penney EB, Pearson J, Dragunow M, Connor B, Faull RL. The distribution of progenitor cells in the subependymal layer of the lateral ventricle in the normal and Huntington's disease human brain. Neuroscience 2005; 132(3):777-788.

[120] Moreno-Lopez B, Romero-Grimaldi C, Noval JA, Murillo-Carretero M, Matarredona ER, Estrada C. Nitric oxide is a physiological inhibitor of neurogenesis in the adult mouse subventricular zone and olfactory bulb. J Neurosci 2004; 24(1):85-95.

[121] Packer MA, Stasiv Y, Benraiss A et al. Nitric oxide negatively regulates mammalian adult neurogenesis. Proc Natl Acad Sci U S A 2003; 100(16):9566-9571.

[122] Pinnock SB, Balendra R, Chan M, Hunt LT, Turner-Stokes T, Herbert J. Interactions between nitric oxide and corticosterone in the regulation of progenitor cell proliferation in the dentate gyrus of the adult rat. Neuropsychopharmacology 2007; 32(2):493-504.

[123] Morrison SJ, Csete M, Groves AK, Melega W, Wold B, Anderson DJ. Culture in reduced levels of oxygen promotes clonogenic sympathoadrenal differentiation by isolated neural crest stem cells. J Neurosci 2000; 20(19):7370-7376.

[124] Studer L, Csete M, Lee SH et al. Enhanced proliferation, survival, and dopaminergic differentiation of CNS precursors in lowered oxygen. J Neurosci 2000; 20(19):7377-7383.

[125] Horie N, So K, Moriya T et al. Effects of oxygen concentration on the proliferation and differentiation of mouse neural stem cells in vitro. Cell Mol Neurobiol 2008; 28(6):833-845.

[126] Galli R, Binda E, Orfanelli U et al. Isolation and characterization of tumorigenic, stem-like neural precursors from human glioblastoma. Cancer Res 2004; 64(19):7011-7021.

[127] Singh SK, Clarke ID, Terasaki M et al. Identification of a cancer stem cell in human brain tumors. Cancer Res 2003; 63(18):5821-5828.

[128] Varghese M, Olstorn H, Sandberg C et al. A comparison between stem cells from the adult human brain and from brain tumors. Neurosurgery 2008; 63(6):1022-1033.

[129] Bao S, Wu Q, McLendon RE et al. Glioma stem cells promote radioresistance by preferential activation of the DNA damage response. Nature 2006; 444(7120):756-760.

[130] Salmaggi A, Boiardi A, Gelati M et al. Glioblastoma-derived tumorospheres identify a population of tumor stem-like cells with angiogenic potential and enhanced multidrug resistance phenotype. Glia 2006; 54(8):850-860.

[131] Visvader JE. Cells of origin in cancer. Nature 2011; 469(7330):314-322.

[132] Alcantara LS, Chen J, Kwon CH et al. Malignant astrocytomas originate from neural stem/progenitor cells in a somatic tumor suppressor mouse model. Cancer Cell 2009; 15(1):45-56.

[133] Marumoto T, Tashiro A, Friedmann-Morvinski D et al. Development of a novel mouse glioma model using lentiviral vectors. Nat Med 2009; 15(1):110-116.

[134] Gibson P, Tong Y, Robinson G et al. Subtypes of medulloblastoma have distinct developmental origins. Nature 2010; 468(7327):1095-1099.

[135] Gage FH. Mammalian neural stem cells. Science 2000; 287(5457):1433-1438.

[136] Erdo F, Buhrle C, Blunk J et al. Host-dependent tumorigenesis of embryonic stem cell transplantation in experimental stroke. J Cereb Blood Flow Metab 2003; 23(7):780-785.

[137] Schwarz SC, Schwarz J. Translation of stem cell therapy for neurological diseases. Transl Res 2010; 156(3):155-160.

[138] Meyer AK, Maisel M, Hermann A, Stirl K, Storch A. Restorative approaches in Parkinson's Disease: which cell type wins the race? J Neurol Sci 2010; 289(1-2):93-103.

[139] Belmonte JC, Ellis J, Hochedlinger K, Yamanaka S. Induced pluripotent stem cells and reprogramming: seeing the science through the hype. Nat Rev Genet 2009; 10(12):878-883.

[140] Levesque F, Neuman T, Rezak M. Therapeutic Microinjection of Autologous Adult Human Neural Stem Cells and Differentiated Neurons for Parkinson's Disease: Five-Year Post-Operative Outcome. The Open Stem Cell Journal 2009; 1:20-29.

[141] Nunes MC, Roy NS, Keyoung HM et al. Identification and isolation of multipotential neural progenitor cells from the subcortical white matter of the adult human brain. Nat Med 2003; 9(4):439-447.

[142] Akesson E, Piao JH, Samuelsson EB et al. Long-term culture and neuronal survival after intraspinal transplantation of human spinal cord-derived neurospheres. Physiol Behav 2007; 92(1-2):60-66.

[143] Varghese M, Olstorn H, Berg-Johnsen J, Moe MC, Murrell W, Langmoen IA. Isolation of human multipotent neural progenitors from adult filum terminale. Stem Cells Dev 2009; 18(4):603-613.

[144] Arvidsson L, Fagerlund M, Jaff N et al. Distribution and Characterization of Progenitor Cells within the Human Filum Terminale. PLoS One 2011; 6(11):e27393.

[145] Sousa-Ferreira L, Alvaro AR, Aveleira C et al. Proliferative hypothalamic neurospheres express NPY, AGRP, POMC, CART and Orexin-A and differentiate to functional neurons. PLoS One 2011; 6(5):e19745.

[146] Murrell W, Feron F, Wetzig A et al. Multipotent stem cells from adult olfactory mucosa. Dev Dyn 2005; 233(2):496-515.

[147] Westerlund U, Svensson M, Moe MC et al. Endoscopically harvested stem cells: a putative method in future autotransplantation. Neurosurgery 2005; 57(4):779-784.

[148] Olstorn H, Moe MC, Roste GK, Bueters T, Langmoen IA. Transplantation of stem cells from the adult human brain to the adult rat brain. Neurosurgery 2007; 60(6):1089-1098.

[149] Sun Y, Pollard S, Conti L et al. Long-term tripotent differentiation capacity of human neural stem (NS) cells in adherent culture. Mol Cell Neurosci 2008; 38(2):245-258.

[150] Walton NM, Sutter BM, Chen HX et al. Derivation and large-scale expansion of multipotent astroglial neural progenitors from adult human brain. Development 2006; 133(18):3671-3681.

[151] Moe MC, Varghese M, Danilov AI et al. Multipotent progenitor cells from the adult human brain: neurophysiological differentiation to mature neurons. Brain 2005; 128(Pt 9):2189-2199.

[152] Moe MC, Westerlund U, Varghese M, Berg-Johnsen J, Svensson M, Langmoen IA. Development of neuronal networks from single stem cells harvested from the adult human brain. Neurosurgery 2005; 56(6):1182-1188.

[153] Westerlund U, Moe MC, Varghese M et al. Stem cells from the adult human brain develop into functional neurons in culture. Exp Cell Res 2003; 289(2):378-383.

[154] Eriksson PS, Perfilieva E, Bjork-Eriksson T et al. Neurogenesis in the adult human hippocampus. Nat Med 1998; 4(11):1313-1317.

[155] Kukekov VG, Laywell ED, Suslov O et al. Multipotent stem/progenitor cells with similar properties arise from two neurogenic regions of adult human brain. Exp Neurol 1999; 156(2):333-344.

[156] Carlen M, Cassidy RM, Brismar H, Smith GA, Enquist LW, Frisen J. Functional integration of adult-born neurons. Curr Biol 2002; 12(7):606-608.

[157] Parent JM, Vexler ZS, Gong C, Derugin N, Ferriero DM. Rat forebrain neurogenesis and striatal neuron replacement after focal stroke. Ann Neurol 2002; 52(6):802-813.

[158] Zhang B, Wang RZ, Yao Y et al. Proliferation and differentiation of neural stem cells in adult rats after cerebral infarction. Chin Med Sci J 2004; 19(2):73-77.

[159] Lichtenwalner RJ, Parent JM. Adult neurogenesis and the ischemic forebrain. J Cereb Blood Flow Metab 2006; 26(1):1-20.

[160] Lindvall O, Kokaia Z. Recovery and rehabilitation in stroke: stem cells. Stroke 2004; 35(11 Suppl 1):2691-2694.

[161] Thored P, Arvidsson A, Cacci E et al. Persistent production of neurons from adult brain stem cells during recovery after stroke. Stem Cells 2006; 24(3):739-747.

[162] Chen J, Li Y, Zhang R et al. Combination therapy of stroke in rats with a nitric oxide donor and human bone marrow stromal cells enhances angiogenesis and neurogenesis. Brain Res 2004; 1005(1-2):21-28.

[163] Curtis MA, Connor B, Faull RL. Neurogenesis in the diseased adult human brain--new therapeutic strategies for neurodegenerative diseases. Cell Cycle 2003; 2(5):428-430.

[164] Jin K, Sun Y, Xie L, Childs J, Mao XO, Greenberg DA. Post-ischemic administration of heparin-binding epidermal growth factor-like growth factor (HB-EGF) reduces infarct size and modifies neurogenesis after focal cerebral ischemia in the rat. J Cereb Blood Flow Metab 2004; 24(4):399-408.

[165] Magavi SS, Leavitt BR, Macklis JD. Induction of neurogenesis in the neocortex of adult mice. Nature 2000; 405(6789):951-955.

[166] Cooper O, Isacson O. Intrastriatal transforming growth factor alpha delivery to a model of Parkinson's disease induces proliferation and migration of endogenous adult neural progenitor cells without differentiation into dopaminergic neurons. J Neurosci 2004; 24(41):8924-8931.

[167] Fallon J, Reid S, Kinyamu R et al. In vivo induction of massive proliferation, directed migration, and differentiation of neural cells in the adult mammalian brain. Proc Natl Acad Sci U S A 2000; 97(26):14686-14691.

[168] Cho SR, Benraiss A, Chmielnicki E, Samdani A, Economides A, Goldman SA. Induction of neostriatal neurogenesis slows disease progression in a transgenic murine model of Huntington disease. J Clin Invest 2007; 117(10):2889-2902.

[169] Kolb B, Gibb R. Brain plasticity and recovery from early cortical injury. Dev Psychobiol 2007; 49(2):107-118.

[170] Cramer SC, Fitzpatrick C, Warren M et al. The beta-hCG+erythropoietin in acute stroke (BETAS) study: a 3-center, single-dose, open-label, noncontrolled, phase IIa safety trial. Stroke 2010; 41(5):927-931.

[171] Park HW, Lim MJ, Jung H, Lee SP, Paik KS, Chang MS. Human mesenchymal stem cell-derived Schwann cell-like cells exhibit neurotrophic effects, via distinct growth factor production, in a model of spinal cord injury. Glia 2010; 58(9):1118-1132.

[172] Tamaki SJ, Jacobs Y, Dohse M et al. Neuroprotection of host cells by human central nervous system stem cells in a mouse model of infantile neuronal ceroid lipofuscinosis. Cell Stem Cell 2009; 5(3):310-319.

[173] Brundin P, Barker RA, Parmar M. Neural grafting in Parkinson's disease Problems and possibilities. Prog Brain Res 2010; 184:265-294.

[174] Freed CR, Greene PE, Breeze RE et al. Transplantation of embryonic dopamine neurons for severe Parkinson's disease. N Engl J Med 2001; 344(10):710-719.

[175] Hagell P, Piccini P, Bjorklund A et al. Dyskinesias following neural transplantation in Parkinson's disease. Nat Neurosci 2002; 5(7):627-628.

[176] Olanow CW, Goetz CG, Kordower JH et al. A double-blind controlled trial of bilateral fetal nigral transplantation in Parkinson's disease. Ann Neurol 2003; 54(3):403-414.

[177] Dihne M, Bernreuther C, Hagel C, Wesche KO, Schachner M. Embryonic stem cell-derived neuronally committed precursor cells with reduced teratoma formation after transplantation into the lesioned adult mouse brain. Stem Cells 2006; 24(6):1458-1466.

[178] Lensch MW, Schlaeger TM, Zon LI, Daley GQ. Teratoma formation assays with human embryonic stem cells: a rationale for one type of human-animal chimera. Cell Stem Cell 2007; 1(3):253-258.

[179] Robinson AJ, Meedeniya AC, Hemsley KM, Auclair D, Crawley AC, Hopwood JJ. Survival and engraftment of mouse embryonic stem cell-derived implants in the guinea pig brain. Neurosci Res 2005; 53(2):161-168.

[180] Kordower JH, Chu Y, Hauser RA, Freeman TB, Olanow CW. Lewy body-like pathology in long-term embryonic nigral transplants in Parkinson's disease. Nat Med 2008; 14(5):504-506.

[181] Li JY, Englund E, Widner H et al. Characterization of Lewy body pathology in 12- and 16-year-old intrastriatal mesencephalic grafts surviving in a patient with Parkinson's disease. Mov Disord 2010; 25(8):1091-1096.

[182] Oya S, Yoshikawa G, Takai K et al. Attenuation of Notch signaling promotes the differentiation of neural progenitors into neurons in the hippocampal CA1 region after ischemic injury. Neuroscience 2009; 158(2):683-692.

[183] Sgubin D, Aztiria E, Perin A, Longatti P, Leanza G. Activation of endogenous neural stem cells in the adult human brain following subarachnoid hemorrhage. J Neurosci Res 2007; 85(8):1647-1655.

[184] Burns TC, Verfaillie CM, Low WC. Stem cells for ischemic brain injury: a critical review. J Comp Neurol 2009; 515(1):125-144.

[185] Miljan EA, Sinden JD. Stem cell treatment of ischemic brain injury. Curr Opin Mol Ther 2009; 11(4):394-403.

[186] Thomas KE, Moon LD. Will stem cell therapies be safe and effective for treating spinal cord injuries? Br Med Bull 2011; 98:127-142.

[187] Falci S, Holtz A, Akesson E et al. Obliteration of a posttraumatic spinal cord cyst with solid human embryonic spinal cord grafts: first clinical attempt. J Neurotrauma 1997; 14(11):875-884.

[188] Wirth ED, III, Reier PJ, Fessler RG et al. Feasibility and safety of neural tissue transplantation in patients with syringomyelia. J Neurotrauma 2001; 18(9):911-929.

[189] Lima C, Pratas-Vital J, Escada P, Hasse-Ferreira A, Capucho C, Peduzzi JD. Olfactory mucosa autografts in human spinal cord injury: a pilot clinical study. J Spinal Cord Med 2006; 29(3):191-203.

[190] Lima C, Escada P, Pratas-Vital J et al. Olfactory mucosal autografts and rehabilitation for chronic traumatic spinal cord injury. Neurorehabil Neural Repair 2010; 24(1):10-22.

[191] http://www.isscr.org/ISSCR_Optimistic_on_Future_of_Stem_Cell_Treatments_Despite_Geron_s_Discontinued_Program.htm

[192] Hyun I, Lindvall O, hrlund-Richter L et al. New ISSCR guidelines underscore major principles for responsible translational stem cell research. Cell Stem Cell 2008; 3(6):607-609.

[193] Lench MW. Public perception of stem cell and genomic research. Genome Medicine 2011; 3:44.

[194] Amariglio N, Hirshberg A, Scheithauer BW et al. Donor-derived brain tumor following neural stem cell transplantation in an ataxia telangiectasia patient. PLoS Med 2009; 6(2):e1000029.

[195] Murrell W, Wetzig A, Donnellan M, Féron F, Burne T, Meedeniya A, Kesby J, Bianco J, Perry C, Silburn P, Mackay-Sim A. Olfactory mucosa is a potential source for autologous stem cell therapy for Parkinson's disease. Stem Cells 2008; 26(8):2183-92

8

An Assistive Surgical MRI Compatible Robot – First Prototype with Field Tests

Tapio Heikkilä[1], Sanna Yrjänä[2], Pekka Kilpeläinen[1],
John Koivukangas[2] and Mikko Sallinen[1]
[1]*VTT Technical Research Centre of Finland*
[2]*Department of Neurosurgery, University of Oulu, Oulu,
Finland*

1. Introduction

1.1 Overview

Magnetic Resonance Imaging (MRI) is superior to other imaging modalities in detecting diseases and pathologic tissue in the human body. The excellent soft tissue contrast allows better delineation of the pathologic and surrounding structures. For example, brain surgery requires exact three-dimensional orientation to piece together anatomical and pathological locations inside the brain. The target location can be seen in the preoperative MRI and neuroradiologists can give assessments, e.g., of tumor nature. Still, factors affecting the resection technique e.g. density of neovasculature and consistency of tumor tissue cannot always be evaluated beforehand. Intraoperative MRI (IMRI) - complementing preoperative MRI – is continuously being developed to give additional information to the neurosurgeon (Tuominen et al., 2002, Yrjänä, 2005).

Robot technology can contribute to working conditions and efficiency of IMRI operations and robots that are compatible with MRI devices represent a new and promising special field in robotics, which can improve clinical diagnostics and treatment for internal diseases, including neurologic ones (Gassert et al., 2008). There are several commercial solutions in operation for surgical robots such as Da Vinci, Minerva, NeuroMate and PathFinder just to mention few but not yet for operation in MRI devices (Zhijiang & Lining, 2003), (Dasgupta & Henderson, 2010), (Jaara, 2007). One solution for assistive surgery is the minimally surgically invasive (MIS) robot which is a large, multi-arm system (Zoppi et. al., 2010). Such kinds of systems are expensive which makes them difficult to reach common use.

1.2 State-of-the-art

Development of MRI compatible robots implies multidisciplinary work. Solutions from conventional robotics are not applicable as such even if the development of such a system is similar to design of a mechatronic device (Cleary & Nguyen, 2001). Strong static and coupling magnetic fields and radio frequency pulses produced by the MRI devices make for a challenging and potentially hazardous environment. Magnetic fields exert forces and eddy currents on materials that are magnetically incompatible or conduct electricity. This may lead to wrong signal information, uncertainties in actuator control and dangerous forces in the construction if they are located in too strong a magnetic field (Virtanen, 2006). Limited working space, limited access to this space, need for line of sight to MR images and comfort of patients and surgeons set additional constraints.

Analysis for optimal design for MRI compatible robots has been proposed by (Gasparetto & Zanotto, 2010). Many MRI compatible robotic devices have also been reported, for biopsies according to the target [for brain (Masamune et al., 1995), breast (Larson et al., 2004), prostate (Susil et. al., 2003)] and also to the structure of the MRI device (Chinzei & Miller, 2001), (Tsekos et al., 2005). To solve the challenge of operation in limited space, a manipulator with several degrees of freedom seems to be best solution, as also proposed in this paper. One solution for that has also been introduced by (Chinzei et. al, 2000). It has good reach by using two manipulator arms but compared to our solution, accuracy is more limited due to lack of efficient calibration. Development of a general purpose device has also been reported (Tsekos et al., 2008).

In comparison, if very high accuracy is needed, also parallel kinematic structures have been presented (Plante et. al., 2009). By constructing the manipulator using dielectric elastomer actuators, here 6 parallel, absolute position accuracy of 1,8mm Root Mean Square (rms) can be reached. Use of this kind of robot structure is limited typically to a volume of a 80x70mm^2 ellipse which limits its use. Operation accuracy has been improved by developing advanced human-robot co-operation where the robot guides the human during the surgery by virtual fixtures which are controlled by using force control, i.e. 6 Degrees-of-Freedom (DOF) force and torque sensor attached to the wrist of the robot (Castillo-Cruces & Wahrburg 2010).

The manipulators developed make use of different methods of actuation, mainly according to four main categories (Elhawary et. al., 2005): transmission by hydraulic or pneumatic actuators, ultrasonic motors based on the piezoceramic principle and remote manual actuation. Progress in materials, position sensing, different actuation techniques, and design strategies have contributed to the technical feasibility in MRI environments, but still most systems lack clinical validation, which is needed for commercial products (Elhawary et. al., 2005), (Gassert et al., 2008). Most advanced example is the NeuroArm (Pandya et al., 2009) which has been developed for open neurosurgical procedures in IMRI environments. NeuroArm is an image-guided, MRI compatible robotic system that is capable of both microsurgery and stereotaxy. However, it is still a manipulator type device where the robot motion control is based on surgeon's manual operations of the joystick type control devices supported by on-line visual information of the MRI device.

Our goal has been a device with portable and readily locatable kinematic structure enabling a variety of applications, like assisting biopsies, tumor operations, and installing automatic dosage implants. Especially requirements from brain surgery, originating from the IMRI guided operations at the Oulu University Hospital (Yrjänä, 2005) have been guiding our work. Semiautomatic operation was targeted where the tool, e.g., a biopsy needle is taken automatically very close to the target location ("entry point"), and final adjustment and needle motions are carried out by the surgeon or at least with tight supervision by the surgeon. The requirement for accuracy of automatic motions is at the level of +/- 1-2 mm for the needle. Finally, we sought to achieve optimal performance within a volume corresponding to that of the human head, our "region of surgical interest" (Koivukangas et al., 2003).

The dimensions of the MRI device and characteristics of the changing magnetic field sets constraints to the robot constructs and dimensions as well as the robot controller hardware (HW), as the robot should not disturb the imaging within IMRI operations, and on the other hand the imaging should not disturb the robot operation. We have developed an MRI compatible robot prototype. MRI compatibility has been introduced in (Virtanen, 2005) and robot control and calibration methods in (Heikkilä et. al, 2009). In the following we give further details about the mechanics, kinematics, calibration, control system and especially results from field tests in the IMRI premises of the Oulu University Hospital. We report to our knowledge on the first robot to repeatedly perform a preprogrammed exercise in the magnetic field of an IMRI scanner in a safe noncollision manner.

2. Mechanical structure and control system

The requirements for the robot prototype were derived based on the experiences of the neurosurgery group at Oulu University Hospital, acquired with IMRI premises with low field horizontally open resistive magnet 0.23 Tesla (T) scanner (Philips, 2011) with a 44 cm patient gap and optical tool navigation devices. During operations while the patient is being imaged, regular operating room products and devices are moved outside a 0.5-mT line (1.5 m from the MR image center point), or out of the imaging room so as not to disturb the imaging (Yrjänä, 2005). The robot controller should be at least outside this 0.5 mT line, or outside the operating room so that the imaging does not induce disturbances to the cables and robot controller HW and vice versa. Correspondingly, the robot main body should be located outside a 2 mT line (1 m from the image center point) to prevent disturbances from imaging to actuators and vice versa.

The MRI compatibility of the robot prototype is designed for the part of the robot which is close to or inside the MRI device during its operation. We have defined, for purposes of neuronavigation (Koivukangas et al., 1993a, b) and robot development, the "region of surgical interest" (ROSI) as the part of the human body that needs to be imaged and then operated using an image guidance method that ensures a suitable minimally invasive surgical approach followed by delineation and treatment of the tumor or other lesion (Koivukangas et al., 2003). Following this principle, our robot has similar kinematic structure as common industrial robots, but with link lengths adjusted to comply with the operation space in the ROSI. The 4th link introduces the needed MRI compatible reach into the working space close to the MR imaging center with its 1000 mm length. The 4th, 5th and 6th links and related joints are made from MRI compatible material, i.e., carbon fiber and aluminium (Virtanen & Nevala, 2007). The bearings in the two last joints are AISI 316 Stainless ball bearings (Virtanen, 2006). The base and the first three links are also made from aluminium.

Joint position sensors for the first four joints are optical encoders and for the last two joints are optical (Harja et al., 2007). The motors are located at the joints, except for the last two joints, for which they are located at the 3rd link with power transmission by nylon strings. The encoder resolutions of the joints were 0.005625 degrees (joint 1), 0.09 degrees (joint 2), 0.09 degrees (joint 3), 0.00625 degrees (joint 4), 0.06 degrees (joint 5), and 0.0125 degrees (joint 6). The repeatability of the tool position (e.g., needle) – as calculated from the encoder resolutions - is at the level of +/- 0.26 mm, +/- 0.24 mm and +/- 0.37 mm in x, y and z directions, respectively. The mechanical outlook of the robot prototype is shown in fig. 1.

wrist motors   carbon fibre MR link   non electric and
                                            non magnetic wrist

joint 4

joint 3

joint 5

joint 6

joint 2

joint 1

aluminum body   shielded electronics

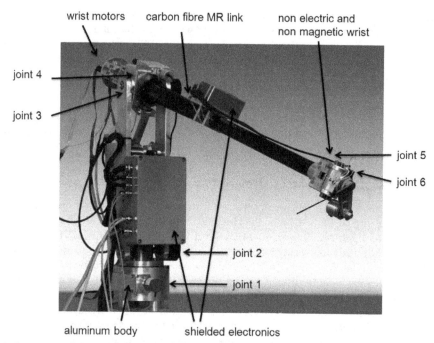

Fig. 1. Structure of the MRI compatible robot prototype.

The working space inside the MRI device is limited and accordingly there are limitations also in the 2nd and 3rd joint motions, +/- 20 degrees and +/- 42 degrees respectively. For other joints the joint limits are looser, i.e. +/- 75 degrees (6th joint) or more. In the wrist there is also a 3 DOF joystick (fig 2.) for the surgeon to control the final adjustment motions. The joystick is made from aluminum and uses fiber-optic sensors (Harja et al., 2007).

biopsy needle   optical joint sensor

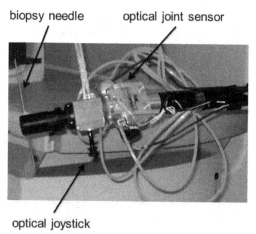

optical joystick

Fig. 2. Optical joystick in the robot wrist

The robot control system is based on a PC/104 controller, with integrated motor drives, and I/O cards for joint measurements and motor controls. The PC/104 controller runs a RT/Linux operating system. The control system is enclosed in RF shielded housing (Rittal Vario-Case iS; fig 3).

The robot control SW is based on RCCL (Robot Control C Library) running on the RT/Linux. The RCCL library [RWRCCL version (Stein, 2004)] implements the joint servo control, trajectory control in joint spaces as well as coordinated motion control in Cartesian space, including inverse kinematic solutions.

RF shielded casing   PC/104 RT Linux PC with I/O cards   Motor drives

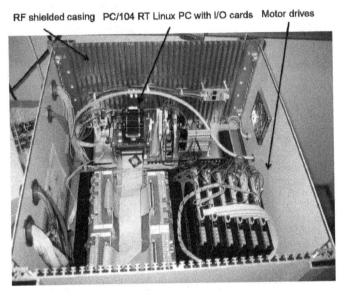

Fig. 3. Control system HW.

3. Work space of assistive surgical tasks

The assistive surgical tasks include presentation of surgical instruments to the surgeon in a proper location with respect to the patient. An exemplary target task goes in two phases:

1. the robot presents the biopsy tool in a proper orientation and location as defined by the surgeon based on the MRI image, and
2. the surgeon carries out the final positioning of the biopsy tool by interactive control, optionally with a redundant axis coincident with the needle axis.

The gross motion paths up to and within the ROSI are carried out by the robot automatically and the fine motions into the contact are guided by the surgeon, either by direct visual feedback from the target or supported by the MRI device. The task space for carrying out the fine motions interactively is limited, and the Cartesian paths of the interactive motions vary little by orientations and a few centimeters by translation.

A simulation model was constructed in the IGRIP simulation tool for studying the paths for brain biopsies in the robot joint space. A simulation model with the MRI compatible robot,

MRI device, and patient is illustrated in fig 4. The robot presents the biopsy tool within a few mm distance from the patients head surface (the "entry point"). In the simulations the nominal interactive paths are following the surface normal of the upper head surface of the patient. In practice the entry point and the target location finally determine the entry orientation.

Because of limitations in the joint motions and the kinematic structure of the robot, the robot base has to be located carefully to avoid singularities in joint space during the interactive motions. With simulations it was confirmed, that a feasible location is on either side of the patient. In other assistive surgical tasks the task space is similar, e.g., above the abdomen.

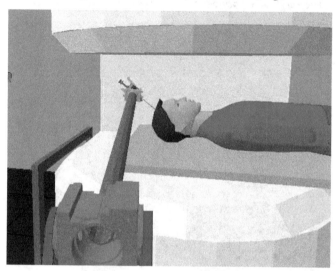

Fig. 4. A feasible entry point location of the MRI compatible robot.

4. Robot calibration

Robot calibration considers internal robot features like joint-axis geometries, joint angle offsets, actuator/link compliances, actuator transmission and coupling factors (Bernhardt & Albright 1993). With precise models for these factors the absolute positioning accuracy can be brought to the level of robot repeatability. Geometric characteristics are concerned by kinematic calibration and kinematic models are usually described by the Denavit-Hartenberg (DH) convention, where the joint axis and link geometry is described as homogeneous transformations with 2 rotational and 2 translational variables. For nominally parallel axis so called modified DH model has been used (Hayati's modified model) with three rotational and 1 translational variable per axis/joint (Zuang & Roth, 1996). The kinematic model is non-linear, and model parameters are typically estimated all at the same time iteratively using the Jacobian of a measurement model. The robot tool positions are recorded together with corresponding joint values and compared to expected positions as calculated by the nominal kinematic model. With linearized error models between the expected and real poses the deviations from the models can be correlated into the form of estimated small corrections, which are added to the nominal parameter values. All independent model parameters can be calculated at the same time and the result is an optimal estimate for the parameter increments with regard to the measurements. Doing this calculation iteratively the parameter values should converge to optimal ones with regard to the measurements.

Another way to estimate the model parameters is to model the joint axis as lines in space and by measuring the robot end point motions while moving joints one-by-one, estimate the axis line models in a joint by joint manner and then calculate the kinematic model parameters from the pairs of estimated line models. The MRI compatible surgery assistant robot operates in very limited joint velocities and it has special geometric structure due to the MRI compatibility requirements – long 3rd link – and so has a special form of work space, which is additionally very limited for the second joint. Considering optimal estimation with all DH parameters estimated at the same time this introduces challenges to compose a proper sample set and fine tune the iterative estimation, e.g., in the Levenberg-Marquardt (LM) form [for details about LM estimation, see, e.g. (Manolis, 2005)]. Because of the robot characteristics and requirements we decided to go for axis-by-axis calibration and compose the DH models for the axis/links subsequently. This resulted in an intuitive calibration procedure and allowed to readily focus on improving sample sets on a joint/axis basis. Although the resulting set of parameter values is not finally optimal, based on extensive simulations it seems satisfactory in the sense of reaching the required kinematic accuracy. It should also be noted, that if finally optimal calibration is required, this kind of sequential axis-by-axis calibration can be used to acquire reliable initial values for truly optimized estimation of the kinematic parameters, e.g., by linearized kinematic models and the LM estimation.

Within the kinematic calibration each joint/link has a local coordinate system attached to the rotating axis. The transformations between the joints and links are modeled following the Denavit-Hartenberg (DH) principle with 2 rotations and 2 translations per axis (rot-trans-trans-rot) with the exception between joints 2 and 3, where modified DH is used (Hayati modification: rot-trans-rot-rot) (Zuang & Roth, 1996). The initial orientations of the local coordinates are here – for our own convenience - slightly different from the original DH convention and are aligned with the base coordinates. The rotations around different joint axes are done as follows: rot-z for the joint 1, rot-x for joints 2,3 and 5, and rot-y for joints 4 and 6 (see fig 5). There are 24 independent parameters, including the transformation from base (world) to the 1st axis and 2nd axis and excluding the tool transformation within the last link.

The calibration is based on observing a point of a calibration target in 3D space while the joint makes a circular motion. Two solutions for measuring the target 3D point were considered: a real multi camera system and a simulated high accuracy laser tracker. The real measurements were carried out with a multi-camera system, where three cameras were located around the working space of the robot (fig 5). Two cameras were located behind the robot with 2 m distance and optical axis towards robot tool and with 90 degrees angles to each other. These were used to observe motions for joints 3, 4, 5 and 6. A third camera was located on the other side of the robot with 1.5 m distance, focusing on motions of joints 1 and 2, and all three cameras were used to observe calibration motions for joints 2 and 3. The voxel accuracies for detecting the calibration target point with Basler Scout scA1400 cameras (1392x1040 pixels) and considering careful camera to camera calibrations, can be estimated to be at the level of +/- 0.5 mm for observing joints 1 and 2, and +/- 1.0 to +/- 1.4 mm for other joints. A fourth camera was used in simulations to test how it can contribute to the calibration accuracy.

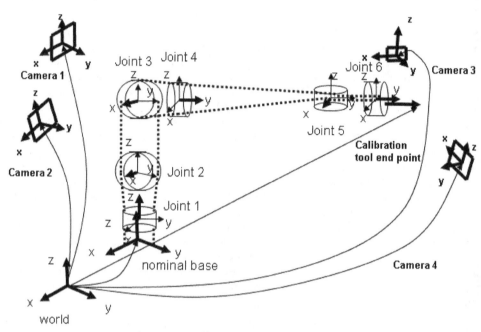

Fig. 5. Overview of the robot joint coordinate systems and a multi-camera system for kinematic calibration measurements

Radial distortion of the lenses was found to be at the level of 0.5 %, and it was corrected in the images before applying image data to the calibrations. The cameras were calibrated to a world frame – and each other – using a flat calibration "world" grid and by estimating the six pose parameters for each camera in the world coordinates. The location of the conic calibration target was measured with different cameras and a corresponding 3D point was constructed based on corrected location in image plane, the pin hole camera model and calibration data (position and orientation) of the cameras.

In the real tests a simple calibration target was observed with the multiple cameras located around the working space of the robot. The image processing routines were simple and based on background lighting and tresholding. This is robust and readily implemented, but repeating precisely same motions (same calibration object locations) will not increase the accuracy in statistical sense. Locating the calibration target object under static lighting conditions results always to a same binary image, because the robot repeatability is much better than the resolution of the camera system.. We added statistical property to the samples by taking three good base positions (fig 6.) for each joint, and added small random variation to the positions. In this way the statistical nature of the samples could be maintained while keeping the best calibration positions, and accuracy improved by increasing the size of sample sets.

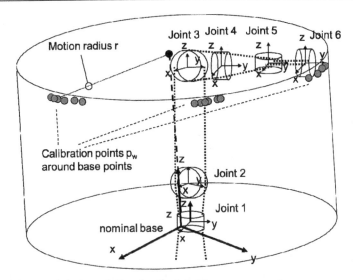

Fig. 6. Base points and their variation for the joint 1 measurements.

The line estimations were done as limited pose estimations, comparable to the pose estimation of paper rolls in (Vähä et al., 1994), with five parameters per joint axis 3D line (2 translation and 2 rotation parameters and the radius of the rotational motion). Jacobians were derived using two fitting criteria: distance of calibration point from the cylindrical surface and distance of calibration point from the plane surface of the rotational motion (circle of the calibration motion). As expected, the convergence in the estimation was in all cases very good, with max 7 to 8 iteration steps. After all the line models for all joints were measured and estimated, the related DH parameters were calculated. Details about the line estimations are given in appendix I and about deriving the DH parameters from the estimated line models are given appendix II.

The sample sets were composed based on the joint motion limits, and the goodness of sample sets was estimated with Matlab simulations. The sizes of sample sets were varied and the tresholding within the voxel accuracy and inaccuracy of the joint servos were taken into consideration; additional white noise ranging with -1, 0 or +1 times the corresponding encoder resolution, was added to the joint values. The simulated sample sizes were 21, 42, 98, and 182 points. In addition, the largest sample set was simulated with a voxel noise corresponding to a more accurate camera (Basler Scout scA1600, with pixel resolution 1628 x 1236) (samples 182/0.75). Simulated results for the DH parameter variation after joint axis estimation are shown in fig 7.

Clearly for all parameters except one it is possible to reach a standard deviation less than 0.1 mm. Bias remains in all parameters independent of the sample sizes; for the translation across the second link axis it is comparably large because of the strict limitation in the joint 2 motions. It was also easily found in the simulations that the bias can be removed if the base points for the axis can be symmetrically spread over the rotation space, with 120 degrees angles between the base points. This is, however, not possible as the joint limits are hard for joints 2, 3, and 5.

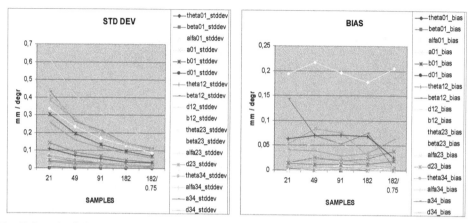

Fig. 7. Standard deviations and bias of the DH parameters

In addition, the tool positioning accuracy was estimated based on the variations of the DH parameters and joint uncertainties (+/- 1 joint encoder pulse). The variation of the end tip location of a biopsy needle (150 mm) was calculated by propagating the covariances of the link/joint transformations from robot base to last link, based on the variances of the DH parameters. Bias was taken as an additive factor to the mean of the corresponding parameters. It was seen, that +/- 1 mm standard deviation is achievable, comparable to +/- 3 mm maximum variation. Lowest estimation accuracy is clearly for the translations parameters between joints 2 and 3, and 3 and 4. The reason is in the limits of the joint 2 motions. The calibration procedure was carried out also with the real robot and a multi-camera system. The results were in expected limits (max deviations from nominal parameter values were less than 1.5 mm), though more thorough testing would give more reliable results and especially details concerning different parameters.

Simulation tests were also carried out using the target tracking accuracy of a Leica Lasertracker (Leica, 2003), for which the absolute measurement accuracy is +/- 0.036 mm. In this case the sample size was 42 points for joints 1 and 2, and 21 points for other joints. The standard deviations were less than 0.08 mm for the translation parameters and 0.0095 degrees for the rotation parameters. Maximum deviations were less than +/- 0.21 mm for the translation parameters and +/- 0.035 degrees for rotation parameters. Cumulative maximum translation deviation was at the level of +/- 0.6 mm for translation parameters, and +/- 0.085 degree for the rotations of the 3 first joints; these are dominating rotations from the point of view of tool locating accuracy because of the long links from the joints up to the tool end tip. This means that with high-end calibration sensors the required kinematic accuracy can readily be achieved.

5. Tests in the IMRI premises

The robot prototype was tested in the 0.23 T intraoperative MRI environment. The used scanner has a C-shaped open configuration with a vertical magnetic field. The premises has been routinely used for neurosurgical operations. The biopsy tool tracking has been achieved using optical 3D tracking devices (Northern Digital, 2011) and registration tags to integrate the patient location and the MR images (Tuominen et al., 2002).

The prototype was fixed to a floor worktop which was set over two props for the tests. Using this arrangement the prototype could be moved to desired points around the scanner. The tests had the following endpoints:

1. Test functionality of the prototype in the magnetic field.
2. Test MR safety and compatibility of the prototype, and
3. Test capability of the robot to move a biopsy needle guide to the correct configuration to allow the surgeon to pass a biopsy needle through the guide to a target

The functionality of the 6 DOF surgical robot was confirmed. It was found capable of positioning an instrument to the desired point and orientation, thus indicating the surgical trajectory from the surface of a target inside the target in the magnetic field. The joystick could be used to move the pointing instrument from the surface of the target inside the target under visual control. Motions of the prototype were fluent except at the margins of the motion ranges (fig. 8).

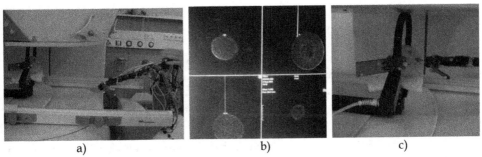

a)   b)   c)

Fig. 8. The surgical robot driven to desired position simulating a biopsy procedure: a) motion towards a target (melon) entry point, b) control view with an custom made optical neuronavigator UI, c) biopsy needle inserted to the target (melon).

The prototype entity was found to be MR safe, but 5th and 6th joints interfered with imaging because of temporarily used incompatible fastener screws. These joints were removed before continuing to the test biopsy. Motors 1 and 4 also malfunctioned when the main body of the robot was within the 20 mT (200 Gauss) fringe field, but the robot could be repositioned to avoid malfunction. All control electronics functioned inside the imaging room but the robot was controlled without displays to minimize electromagnetic noise. The keyboard caused disturbances and needed to be turned off during imaging. Servo motors caused some noise in the MR images despite the EMC shielding box.

The capability of the prototype to pass a biopsy needle guide to a correct configuration was tested with a melon (cucumis melo) fixed to an intraoperative RF coil integrated head holder A fatty vitamin capsule was inserted inside the melon before it was placed for the MR imaging and scanned using a fast field echo imaging sequence. The needle guide was fixed to a 10 cm long extension piece which was applied to the robot arm in place of the 5th and 6th joints. The robot prototype was then programmed to drive the needle guide to a distance 10 mm from the surface of the melon. The tip of the biopsy needle was driven into correct position first using the joystick controls. The robot was then programmed to repeat a series of non-collision steps to reposition the needle correctly to aforementioned position. The actual biopsy procedure was then simulated by passing the biopsy needle by hand through the guide until the tip of the needle hit the vitamin capsule inside the melon. A tag of the optical tool tracking system was connected to the biopsy needle and the tool tracking was used to guide and verify the insertion successfully, including the entry and final locations of the needle tip inside the melon (fig 8 b).

6. Discussion

A working readily maneuverable robot prototype has been constructed. The working space is generally limited, but suitable for IMRI related operations in the region of surgical interest. Motion control based on the RCCL library was quick to implement and was easily used as far as robots paths needed to be programmed. Because the Cartesian speed of a tool (e.g., a biopsy needle) can be very low (ca. 5 cm / sec), the feasibility of joint trajectories has been achieved in test runs.

The kinematic calibration was carried out in a simple and straightforward way. The limitations of joints, especially for joint 2, clearly caused the largest estimation uncertainties in the related DH parameters. Based on simulations the required accuracy is still achievable if the laser tracker is used for tracking the calibration target. A multi camera system can be used as well, but usability with the ordinary cameras we have been using is limited for cross checking the kinematic parameter values. Still, for interactive control of fine motions with tight integration of the surgeon this is enough. For more advanced automatic motion control the remaining uncertainties would require laser tracker based calibration.

From the presented ROSI principle it follows, that the surgical guidance device must be optimized for functionality in the volume of the ROSI, which in neurosurgery means that of the human head. This involves dividing the tasks of the robot into gross and local movements. This was achieved in the present tests by robotic movement of the needle guide to a predetermined position 10 mm from the target followed by manual passage of the needle to the target.

The longer term goal is to integrate the robot and its usage tighter with MR images. This will lead to integration of the MRI device with respect to the robot coordinate system and then using the same technology for tracking the tool attached to the robot end tip. This will substantially loosen the accuracy requirements of the robot: global accuracy will be taken care by the optical tracking tool [currently at the level of +/- 0.7 mm (Katisko, 2007)] after which local accuracy of the robot becomes critical, just like in the case of interactive control. It is also noteworthy that there are varying IMRI practices for imaging and operating, e.g., the following (Yrjänä, 2005):

- Imager lowered for surgery
- Surgery in fringe field
- Surgery in adjacent Operation Room
- Magnetic field turned off for surgery
- Surgery in imaging space
- Surgery adjacent to the imaging space
- Imager moved away for surgery

Depending on the case, the requirements for the robot may vary quite much. We have reached the level of a prototype principally compatible with the IMRI premises and optimized for the ROSI. However, the varying imaging and operating practices create challenges for deciding the next stages of development.

The present robot project was a logical continuation in our research community of early experience with the development of neuronavigation based on a 6 DOF passive mechatronic arm (Koivukangas et al., 1993a, b). This device was routinely clinically used for image-guided procedures, guiding a variety of instruments in the same way as optical tracking systems. The mechatronic arm had joints that were designed to house both electromagnetic clutch brakes and servo motors.

The rationale for developing an active robot arose from the need to transfer the result of presurgical planning directly to the surgical field, like by the Robodoc (Bargar et. al. 1998), which can be preprogrammed to create an optimal boney fit for prostheses in hip and knee replacement surgery. From the other reported IMRI developments the present robot differs in that it was specified to perform safe preprogrammed movement of a needle guide to the target in the region of surgical interest and to act as a stative, or needle guide holder, while the surgeon passes the biopsy needle or forceps to the target--all of this in the magnetic field of an IMRI scanner. It was a necessary first step to confirm the functionality and accuracy of our robotic solution. With continued experience in both robotics and image-guided surgery, our group plans on extending the functionality of the robot.

7. Conclusions

A prototype robot for assisting surgery operations in IMRI environments was described in this paper. We reported on the robot to repeatedly perform a preprogrammed exercise in the magnetic field of an IMRI scanner in a safe noncollision manner. The target was a fatty vitamin pill placed inside a melon. The robot brought the end effector into the region of surgical interest and positioned the tip of the needle guide holder 10 mm from the object, serving as a stereotactic device to enable the passage of the biopsy instrument to its exact final target.

The mechatronic structure, calibration and experimental tests in an IMRI environment were explained in more details. Simulations showed that expected locating accuracy from the point of view of joint sensors and calibrations sensors can be achieved. The robot could be operated in a semiautomatic manner, either running paths or interactively using joystick, in joint space or Cartesian space. Field tests in the hospital IMRI unit confirmed the applicability of the system in the region of surgical interest even under MRI conditions.

8. Appendix I: Estimation of the axis as a line in space

The calibration is carried out in a joint by joint manner. Each joint is moved one by one, and the end tip 3D coordinates of the calibration object is recorded in world frame. For each joint motion a 3D line model of the joint is calculated, which results to six 3D line models in the world frame. From these line models the DH parameters are further calculated.

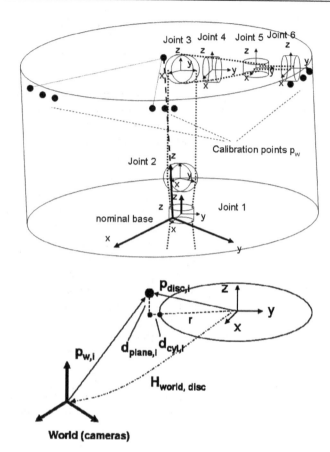

The robot makes a rotary calibration motion around the calibrated axis, where the measured end point of the arm tip forms a "disc" in space. Then the parameters of the calibrated axis are given as a pose $\overline{H}_{world,disc}$ which is presented in a homogeneous matrix form in zyx Euler form:

$$\overline{p}_{i,disc} = \overline{H}_{world,disc} * \overline{p}_{i,world}$$

for which

$$\overline{H}_{world,disc} = f\left(\overline{\theta}\right)$$

Let the state vector $\overline{\theta}_{all}$ all be composed of the parameters of the calibrated axis and related calibration data:

$$\overline{\theta}_{all} = \begin{bmatrix} \overline{\theta} & r \end{bmatrix}$$

where

θ is the vector of pose parameters and,

r is the radius of the rotation "disc", i.e., around the axis.

The pose parameters of the "disc" are then

$$\bar{\theta} = \begin{bmatrix} \alpha & \beta & \chi & x & y & z \end{bmatrix}^T$$

where

a is rotation around x axis,

β is rotation around y axis

χ is rotation around z axis, here undefined,

x is x coordinate,

y is y coordinate,

z is z coordinate,

We have nominal values for the "disc" pose parameters, to which the measured 3D points are matched. Because the rotational part of the "disc" pose are non-linear, we define two error measures, related to which we linearize the measurement model.

Let the error measure for point i be

$$\bar{e}_i = \begin{bmatrix} d_{plane,i} \\ d_{cyl,i} \end{bmatrix}$$

where $d_{plane,i}$ is distance from the measured point to the disc plane and

$d_{cyl,i}$ is distance from the measured point to the cylindrical surface set by the disc

The nominal disc location is always in origin, so the distance from the measured point to the disc plane is the z coordinate of the measured point in the disc pose:

$$d_{plane} = \bar{p}_{disc,z}$$

The distance from the cylindrical surface of the disc is in a similar way

$$d_{cyl} = \sqrt{p_{s,disc,x}^2 + p_{s,disc,y}^2} - r$$

Now we derive the linear relationship between the error measure and the state parameters:

$$\frac{\partial \bar{e}}{\partial \bar{\theta}} = \frac{\partial \bar{e}}{\partial \bar{p}_{disc}} * \frac{\partial \bar{p}_{disc}}{\partial \bar{\theta}}$$

for which

$$\frac{\partial d_{plane}}{\partial \bar{p}_{disc}} = \frac{\partial \bar{p}_{disc,z}}{\partial \bar{p}_{disc}} = \begin{bmatrix} 0 & 0 & 1 \end{bmatrix}$$

and

$$\frac{\partial d_{cyl}}{\partial \overline{p}_{disc}} = \left[\frac{p_{disc,x}}{\sqrt{p_{s,disc,x}^2 + p_{s,disc,y}^2}} \quad \frac{p_{disc,y}}{\sqrt{p_{s,disc,x}^2 + p_{s,disc,y}^2}} \quad 0 \right]$$

The partial derivatives of the measured point in the disc pose are

$$\frac{\partial \overline{p}_{disc}}{\partial \theta} = \begin{bmatrix} 0 & p_{disc,z} & -p_{disc,y} & 1 & 0 & 0 \\ -p_{disc,z} & 0 & p_{disc,x} & 0 & 1 & 0 \\ p_{disc,y} & -p_{disc,x} & 0 & 0 & 0 & 1 \end{bmatrix}$$

The 3rd column will be omitted, because the rotation around the calibrated axis, i.e., around the z-axis of the disc pose cannot be estimated.

For the radius of the disc we get

$$\frac{\partial d_{cyl}}{\partial r} = -1$$

Finally the estimate the parameter increments for the updated 6 parameters (rotation around z axis omitted):

$$\Delta \overline{\theta} = \begin{pmatrix} \Delta \alpha \\ \Delta \beta \\ \Delta x \\ \Delta y \\ \Delta z \\ \Delta r \end{pmatrix} = -\left(\overline{J}^T * \overline{J} \right)^{-1} * \overline{J}^T * \overline{e}$$

where the Jacobian

$$\overline{J} = \frac{\partial \overline{e}}{\partial \overline{\theta}}$$

The complete estimation algorithm is as follows:

0. set initial disc pose and radius
1. calculate nominal calibration point positions in disc frame
2. calculate error measures for each calibration point
3. calculate the Jacobian, i.e., the partial derivatives
6. calculate parameters increments for the state parameters
7. update the state parameters
8. if increments not 'small enough', go to 1, otherwise end.

9. Appendix II: From line models to DH parameters

Measured axis lines are given as an arbitrary point in the line p_i and a normalized direction vector n_i. From a pair of these the DH parameters or modified DH parameters will be derived.

DH parameters

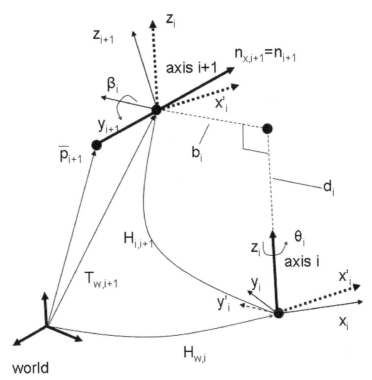

Transformation from the joint i coordinates to joint $i+1$ coordinates goes, according to the DH parameters, in four steps:

- rotate H_i around z_i with θ_i so that x_{i+1} aligns with the zx_i plane
- transfer H_i along z_i with d_i to a point where distance from x_{i+1} is shortest
- transfer H_i along y_i with b_i to an intersection point with x_{i+1}
- rotate H_i around y_i with β_i so that x_{i+1} aligns with x_i

The transformation from world/base coordinates, in which the lines are measured, to the local coordinates of joint I can be divided to rotation and translation parts:

$$H_{w,i} = \begin{bmatrix} \overline{R}_{w,i} & \overline{T}_{w,i} \end{bmatrix}$$

For the rotation between the joint coordinates i and $i+1$ we start from the unit vectors of the transformation.

$$R_{i,i+1} = \begin{bmatrix} \overline{n}_{x,i,i+1} & \overline{n}_{y,i,i+1} & \overline{n}_{z,i,i+1} \end{bmatrix}$$

Unit vector of x is aligned with the axis of joint $i+1$, and so we can derive the unit vectors for y and z:

$$\overline{n}_{y,i+1} = \frac{\overline{n}_{z,i} \times \overline{n}_{x,i+1}}{\left\| \overline{n}_{z,i} \times \overline{n}_{x,i+1} \right\|}$$

$$\overline{n}_{z,i+1} = \overline{n}_{x,i+1} \times \overline{n}_{y,i+1}$$

Axis of joint $i+1$, i.e., $n_{x,i+1}$ in joint i coordinates is then

$$\overline{n}_{x,i+1,i} = \overline{H}_{w,i}^{-1} * \overline{n}_{x,i+1}$$

and as coordinates

$$\overline{n}'_{x,i+1,i} = \begin{bmatrix} x_{n,x,i+1,i} \\ y_{n,x,i+1,i} \\ z_{n,x,i+1,i} \end{bmatrix}$$

Then we get for the angle θ_i

$$\theta_i = a\tan(\frac{y_{n,x,i+1,i}}{x_{n,x,i+1,i}})$$

and for the angle β_i

$$\beta_i = -a\sin(z_{n,x,i+1,i})$$

For the translation in direction of $y_{i,i+1}$ we get the same as the distance b_i between the axis i and axis i+1:

The point of axis $i+1$ after rotation by θ_i as $H_{i,\theta}$

$$\overline{H}_{\theta,i} = \begin{bmatrix} \cos(\theta) & -\sin(\theta) & 0 & 0 \\ \sin(\theta) & \cos(\theta) & 0 & 0 \\ 0 & 0 & 1 & 0 \\ 0 & 0 & 0 & 1 \end{bmatrix}$$

and

$$\overline{P}_{1,i,i+1} = \overline{H}_{w,i}^{-1} * \overline{H}_{\theta,i}^{-1} * \overline{P}_{1,w,i+1}$$

Then we get

$$b_i = \overline{P}_{i,i+1,y}$$

Axis $i+1$ is located in the direction of the rotated xz plane, with the distance of b_i from this plane. The point in axis $i+1$ which is closest to axis i is also located in rotated yz plane. From point p this closest point locates to the direction of x_{i+1} with the following coefficient

$$k = -\frac{p_{i,i+1,x}}{n_{x,i,i+1}}$$

and then the point gets the z coordinate and also the translation along the z-axis of $H_{w,i}$ as

$$d_i = p_{i,i+1,z} + k * z_{nxi,i+1}$$

Modified DH parameters

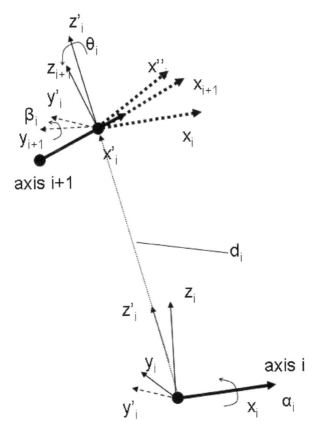

Transformation from the joint i coordinates to joint $i+1$ coordinates goes, according to the modified DH parameters, in four steps:

- rotation around x axis i with a_i to direct z axis towards axis $i+1$
- translation of H_i with d_i to intersect the axis $i+1$
- rotate around z with θ_i and
- rotate around y with β_i so that the coordinate systems are aligned

The distance of the point of axis *i+1* in the *zy* plane of the frame H_i is the *x* coordinate of point p_{i+1} in the axis *i+1*. The intersection point of the axis *i+1* with the *zy* plane – and the origin of the frame H_{i+1} becomes then

$$H_{w,i} = \begin{bmatrix} \bar{R}_{w,i} & \bar{T}_{w,i} \end{bmatrix}$$

For the translation between the joint coordinate systems we get

$$\bar{T}_{i,i+1} = \bar{P}_{i,i+1} + \frac{P_{i,i+1,x}}{n_{i,i+1,x}} * \bar{n}_{i,i+1}$$

and the rotation angle a_i becomes then

$$\alpha_{i,i+1} = a\tan\left(\frac{T_{i,i+1,y}}{T_{i,i+1,z}}\right)$$

The link transformation after rotation a_i becomes then

$$\bar{H}_{a,i} = \begin{bmatrix} 1 & 0 & 0 & T_{i,i+1,x} \\ 0 & \cos(\alpha) & -\sin(\alpha) & T_{i,i+1,y} \\ 0 & \sin(\alpha) & \cos(\alpha) & T_{i,i+1,z} \\ 0 & 0 & 0 & 1 \end{bmatrix}$$

and further

$$\bar{H}_{a,i} = \begin{bmatrix} \bar{R}_{i,i+1,\alpha} & \bar{T}_{i,i+1} \\ 0 \quad 0 \quad 0 & 1 \end{bmatrix}$$

where

$$\bar{R}_{i,i+1,\alpha} = \begin{bmatrix} \bar{n}_{x,i,i+1,\alpha} & \bar{n}_{y,i,i+1,\alpha} & \bar{n}_{z,i,i+1,\alpha} \end{bmatrix}$$

For the *y* and *z* axis for the frame H_{i+1} we get then

$$\bar{n}_{y,i+1} = \frac{\bar{n}_{z,i,i+1,\alpha} \times \bar{n}_{x,i+1}}{\left\| \bar{n}_{z,i,i+1,\alpha} \times \bar{n}_{x,i+1} \right\|}$$

$$\bar{n}_{z,i+1} = \bar{n}_{x,i+1} \times \bar{n}_{y,i+1}$$

The direction vector of the axis *i+1* becomes after the rotation a_i around *x* axis *i*

$$\bar{n}_{1,i,i+1,\alpha} = \bar{H}_{a,i}^{-1} * \bar{n}_{i,i+1}$$

The rotation angle θ_i around z axis is then

$$\theta_{i,i+1} = a\tan\left(\frac{n_{i,i+1,\alpha,y}}{n_{i,i+1,\alpha,x}}\right)$$

The link transformation after rotation θ_i becomes then

$$\overline{H}_{\alpha,\theta,i} = \overline{H}_{\alpha,i} * \overline{H}_{\theta,i}$$

where

$$\overline{H}_{\theta,i} = \begin{bmatrix} \cos(\theta) & -\sin(\theta) & 0 & 0 \\ \sin(\theta) & \cos(\theta) & 0 & 0 \\ 0 & 0 & 1 & 0 \\ 0 & 0 & 0 & 1 \end{bmatrix}$$

The transformation can be given also with the rotation and translation parts

$$\overline{H}_{\alpha,\theta,i} = \begin{bmatrix} \overline{R}_{i,i+1,\alpha,\theta,i} & T_{i,j+1} \\ 0 \;\; 0 \;\; 0 & 1 \end{bmatrix}$$

where

$$\overline{R}_{i,i+1,\alpha,\theta} = \begin{bmatrix} \overline{n}_{x,i,i+1,\alpha,\theta} & \overline{n}_{y,i,i+1,\alpha,\theta} & \overline{n}_{z,i,i+1,\alpha,\theta} \end{bmatrix}$$

Finally the rotation angle β_i around y axis is

$$\beta_{i,i+1} = -a\tan\left(\frac{n_{i,i+1,\alpha,\theta,z}}{n_{i,i+1,\alpha,\theta,x}}\right)$$

10. Acknowledgements

The Oulu medical robotics community has over 20 years of experience in the field of medical applications, and some earlier contributions of it are also referred to in the text. The authors would like to acknowledge many colleagues who contributed to the realization of the robot prototype: Yrjö Louhisalmi LicTech (ME), Prof. Kalervo Nevala PhD (ME), Jani Virtanen PhD, Jani Katisko LicTech (biophysics), Pekka Isto PhD, Tapani Koivukangas MS (ME), Pirkka Tukeva MS (ME), Matti Annala engineer, and Jari Hämeenaho technician.

11. References

Bargar W. L., Bauer A., Börner M. Primary and revision total hip replacement using the Robodoc system. Clin Orthop Relat Res. 1998, Sep;(354):82-91.

Bernhardt R. & Albright S. (1993). Introduction. In Bernhardt R., Albright S (eds.): *Robot Calibration*, Chapman & Hall, Cambridge 1993, 311 p.

Castillo-Cruces R. & Wahrburg J. (2010). Virtual fixtures with autonomous error compensation for human-robot cooperative tasks. *Robotica* (2010) Vol 28, 2, pp. 267-277.

Chinzei K. & Miller K. (2001). MRI guided surgical robot, In: *Proceedings of the Australian Conference of Robotics and Automation*, Sydney 2001, pp. 50–55.

Chinzei K., Hata N., Jolesz F.A., Kikinis R. (2000). MR Compatible Surgical Assist Robot: System Integration and Preliminary Feasibility Study. In: *Proceedings of the 3rd International Conferece of Medical Image Computing and Computer-Assisted Intervention*, Pittsburg, Pennsylvenia, USA, 11-14 October. 2000; pp. 921-930.

Cleary K. & Nguyen C. (2001). State of the Art in Surgical Robotics: Clinical Applications and Technology Challenges. *Computer Aided Surgery*, November 2001. 26p

Dasgupta P., Henderson A., (2010). Robotic urological surgery. *Robotica* (2010) Vol 28, pp. 235-240.

Elhawary H., Zivanovic A., Davies B. & Lamperth M. (2005), A review of magnetic resonance imaging compatible manipulators in surgery. *Proceedings of IMechE*, Vol. 220 Part H: Journal of Engineering in Medicine, pp. 413 - 424.

Gasparetto A., Zanotto V. (2010). Toward an optimal performance index for neurosurgical robot's design. *Robotica* (2010) Vol 28, pp. 279-296

Gassert R., Burdet E, & Chinzei K. (2008). MRI-Compatible Robotics. A Critical Tool for Image-Guided Interventions, Clinical Diagnostics, and Neuroscience. *IEEE Engineering in in Medicine and Biology Magazine*, May/June 2008, pp. 12 - 14.

Harja J., Tikkanen J., Sorvoja H. & Myllylä, R. (2007). Magnetic resonance imaging-compatible, three-degrees-of-freedom joystick for surgical robot. *The International Journal of Medical Robotics and Computer Assisted Surgery*, Vol.3, Issue 4, (December 2007), 7 p.

Heikkilä T., Isto P., Järviluoma M., Kilpeläinen P., Sallinen M. (2009). A Prototype for an Assistive Surgical MRI Compatible Robot. *The 14th IASTED International Conference on Robotics and Applications - RA 2009*. November 4 - 6, 2009, Cambridge, Massachusetts, USA.

Jaara J. (2007). *Designing surgical robot for clinical robot for MR-imaging environment.* Diploma thesis, University of Oulu (in finnish). 60p + 12p appendixes.

Katisko J & Koivukangas J (2007) Optically neuronavigated ultrasonography in an intraoperative magnetic resonance imaging environment. *Neurosurgery* 60(4 Suppl 2): 373–381.

Koivukangas J., Louhisalmi Y., Alakuijala J., Oikarinen J. (1993a) Ultrasound-controlled neuronavigator-guided brain surgery. *J Neurosurg* 79: 36-42.

Koivukangas J., Louhisalmi Y., Alakuijala J., Oikarinen J. (1993b) Neuronavigator-guided cerebral biopsy. *Acta Neurochir Suppl* 58: 71-74.

Koivukangas J, Katisko J, Yrjänä S, Tuominen J, Schiffbauer H, Ilkko E (2003) Successful neurosurgical 0.23T intraoperative MRI in a shared facility. *Neurosurgery* 2003. Monduzzi Editore Medimond: 439-444.

Larson B. T., Erdman A. G., Tsekos N. V., Yacoub E., Tsekos P. V. & Koutlas I. G. (2004). Design of an MRI-compatible robotic stereotactic device for minimally invasive interventions in the breast, *Journal of Biomechanical Engineering*, vol. 126, pp. 458–465.

Leica Geosystems (2003). *Leica Absolute Tracker™ With PowerLock Active Vision Technology*. Available from http://www.leica-geosystems.com/en/Laser-Tracker-Systems-Leica-Absolute-Tracker_69047.htm

Manolis I. (2005). A. A brief description of the Levenberg-Marquardt algorithm implemented by levmar. *Foundation for research and technology*, Heraklion, 2005.

Masamune, K., Kobayashi E., Masutani Y., Suzuki M., Dohi T., Iseki H. & Takakura K.(1995). Development of an MRI-compatible needle insertion manipulator for stereotactic neurosurgery. *Journal of Image Guided Surgery*, vol. 1, pp. 242–248.

Northern Digital Inc. (2011). *Polaris Family of Optical Tracking Systems*. Available from: http://www.ndigital.com/medical/polarisfamily.php

Ojala, R. (2002). *MR-guided interventions at 0.23T. Facilities, user interface, guiding technology and musculoskeletal applications*. PhD Thesis, University of Oulu, 73 p.

Pandya S., Motkoski J. W., Serrano-Almeida C., Greer A. D., Latour I., Sutherland G. R., Advancing Neurosurgery with Image-Guided Robotics. *Journal of Neurosurgery* 111:1141-1149, 2009.

Philips, Panorama 0.23T R/T Manufacturer Specifications (2011). Available from http://www.medwow.com/med/mri/philips/panorama-0-23t-r-t/28837.model-spec

Plante J-S., Lauren M., DeVita K., Kacher D., Roebuck J., DiMaio S., Jolesz F. & Dubowsky S. An MRI-Compatible Needle Manipulator Concept Based on Elastically Averaged Dielectric Elastomer Actuators for Prostate Cancer Treatment: An Accuracy and MR-Compatibility Evaluation in Phantoms. *Journal of Medical Devices*, Sep. 2009, Vol 3. 10p.

Stein, M. (2004). RWRCCL: *A New RCCL Implementation Using Real-Time Linux And A Single CPU*. Available from: http://faculty.rwu.edu/mstein/verbiage/RWRCCL.pdf

Susil R. C., Krieger A., Derbyshire J. A., Tanacs A., Whitcomb L. L., Fichtinger G. & Atalar E. (2003). System for MR image-guided prostate interventions: Canine study, *Radiology*, vol. 228, pp. 886–894.

Tsekos N. V., Ozcan A. & Christoforou E. (2005). A prototype manipulator for MR-guided interventions inside standard cylindrical MRI scanners. *Journal of Biomechanical Engineering*, vol. 127, pp. 972–980.

Tsekos N., Christoforou E. & Özcan, A. (2008). A General-Purpose MR-Compatible Robotic System - Implementation and Image Guidance for Performing Minimally Invasive Interventions. *IEEE in Engineering and Biology Magazine*, May/June 2008, pp. 51 - 58.

Tuominen, J., Yrjänä S. K., Katisko J. P., Heikkilä J., Koivukangas J (2002) Intraoperative imaging in a comprehensive neuronavigation environment for minimally invasive brain tumor surgery. *Acta Neurochir Suppl* 85: 115-120.

Virtanen, J. (2006). *Enhancing the compatibility of surgical robots with magnetic resonance imaging*. PhD Thesis, University of Oulu, 2006. 196 p.

Virtanen, J. & Nevala, K. (2007). MR- compatibility of an intraoperative robot. *12th IFToMM Word Congress*, Besancon, France, June 18-21, 2007. 6 p.

Vähä P., Heikkilä T., Röning J. & Okkonen J. (1994). Machine of the Future: An Intelligent Paper Roll Manipulator. *Mechatronics*, Vol. 4, No. 8, pp. 861 - 877.

Yrjänä S. (2005). *Implementation of 0.23 T magnetic resonance scanner to perioperative imaging in neurosurgery*. PhD Thesis, University Of Oulu, 2005, 71 p.

Zhijiang D., Lining S. Review of Surgical Robotics and Key Technologies Analysis. In: *Proceedings of the IEEE International Conference on Robotics, Intelligent Systems and Signal Processing*. Changsha, China, October 2003, pp. 1041 – 1046.

Zoppi M., Khan M., Schäfer F., Molfino R. (2010). Toward lean minimally invasive robotic surgery. *Robotica* (2010) Vol 28, pp. 185-197.

Zuang H. & Roth Z. (1996). *Camera-Aided Robot Calibration*. CRC Press Inc., Florida, USA, 1996, 353 p.

Section 4

Appendix

9

Hemostatic Agents in Neurosurgery

F. Lapierre, S. D'Houtaud and M. Wager

1. Introduction

Adequate hemostasis is a prerequisite in neurosurgery, to prevent dramatic postoperative bleedings and their consequences. Different sorts of local hemostatic agents have been developed, with a variable efficacy. Some of them have been used for years, none being perfect.

The residual presence of these agents may behave as foreign bodies, and induce inflammation, infection, and even delayed bone growth.

Safety is an other concern since most of modern agents contain more or less human and animal components.

We are going to review the history of those agents, their different categories, compare them and try to establish some guidelines when using them, with their different indications.

2. Hemostasis (basis)

Hemostasis comes from the coordinated activation of platelets and plasma clotting factors to form a platelet fibrin clot. Two processes, primary and secondary hemostasis activation of the clotting cascade id done by collagen for the intrinsic pathway, and the extrinsic pathway is activated by the release of tissue factors from the damaged zone. The two converge ento the common pathway which begins with the conversion of Factor X to Xa, the conversion of prothrombin to thrombin, which is integral in clot stabilization via fibrin. This common pathway is facilitated by Factor V (Hawiger 1987).

3. History

From the beginning of the neurosurgical practice, local hemostatic agents have proved to be very useful completing the more classical use of the electrocoagulation whatever its type, mono or bipolar or sometimes laser.

3.1 First attempts

3.1.1 Auto or hetero-muscle application

Until the early 1950, neurosurgeons used as topical hemostatic agents fresh chicken breast which was delivered to the operative theatre just before the beginning of the operation. Electrocoagulation device was not very good, and they often had to apply the chicken flesh on the brain during ten minutes while washing the field with warm serum, and removed it before closing the dura.

Fresh muscle harvested from the temporal site or the thigh is still commonly used for extradural dural hemostasis and may be left in situ.

At the same times, bone wax was used and is still used for bone hemostasis (Grant 2007). Bone wax was created by Sir Victor Haden Horsley (1857-1916) from beewax in 1892. Since this period different components were added to wax, but the common name remained "Horsley wax".

3.2 Hydrogen peroxide

It has been used for decades as a hemostatic agent and is believed to establish hemostasis through its vasoconstrictive properties, and is also credited to create a disruption of the blood-barrier and an aggregation of the platelets and neutrophils leading to thrombus formation. The free diffusion of H2O2 through the vessel walls and its conversion to water and 02 leads to intra-luminal bubbles, micro-embolisms and vessels obstruction.

3.3 Modern evolution

Multiple local hemostatic agents now exist (Abaut & Basle 2003, Grant 2007)

3.3.1 Fibrin sealants

The better understanding of hemostasis mechanisms brought new perspectives for the conception of other local agents. The first discussion for topical agents is due to Bergen who emphasized the role of fibrin in hemostasis. Secundary, this will move to the preparation of fibrin sealants, the first combination of bovine thrombin with human plasma for topical use. In 1938, purified thrombin became available, with obtention of new fibrin sealants used in 1940, as reported in the literature, even for nerve repair. In 1944, their use was reported to optimize skin-grafts survival and adhesion of skin grafts, in severe burn injury during the war by Cronkite. Richard Upjohn Light 1945 reviews the different existing helps to improve hemostasis in neurosurgery, and Fincher 1946 reports the uses of gelatin foam .

But the technics used in those times only led to preparations being the potential source of transmission of viral hepatitis. So bovine thrombin was substituted for human thrombin to minimize the risk of viral transmission. But some patients developed coagulopathies due to the use of bovine thrombin related to immune-mediated production of thrombin and factorV inhibitors.

All these difficulties led to abandon the fibrin sealants for years.

In the late 1960, isolation and concentration of clotting factors from human plasma became possible, and in 1972, Matras produced the first item of modern fibrin sealants. The first commercially fibrin sealant was approved in Europe in 1982, and Later in USA in 1990.

In 1998, Tisseel and Hemascel sealants were approved by FDA, and the firs sealant with entirely human components called Crosseals was made in 1993. Surgical use widely spread in nearly all specialities.

3.3.2 Gelatin hemostatic agents

They were introduced in 1940 such as Gelfoam and Surgifoam.

Gelfoam is a purified pork skin gelatine with hemostatic properties which may come from its physical features, and not from an effect on the clotting cascade. It may be used with saturated thrombin.

They exist as sponges and have a capacity to expand up to 200% in vivo, which may be a negative property in some deep fields specially in neurosurgery.

Floseal combines human derived thrombin with bovine derived gelatin matrix granules which are mixed at the time of use, and also exists as a liquid device minimizing the expansion property, allowing its application in minimal invasive surgery and neurosurgery.

3.3.3 Cyanoacrylate adhesives

They were developed by Dr H Coover in 1942. It consists cyanoacrylate monomers which polymerize in long chains in the presence of hydroxyl ions.

3.3.4 Oxyfied regenerated glucose

Is a plant –based topical hemostatic introduced in 1960. It is made by regenerating a pure plant-derived cellulose secondary knitted and oxidized. It acts as a scaffold for clot formation. On post-operative imaging, it may mimic an abcess or some residual tumor.

3.3.5 Microfibrillar collagen

This substance (Avitene) was introduced in 1970. Microfibrillar applied collagen products come from the purification of bovine collagen, followed by microcristallisation. It is presented as a powder, and is more effective than gelatine based hemostasis, since it is able to activate the clotting cascade.

3.4 Thrombin and fibrinogen (fibrin glue)

Are the most recently appeared.

Fibrin glues contain thrombin and fibrinogen: when combined, the fibrinogen is activated by thrombin and converted into fibrin monomere which form an adhesive glue at the tissues applied.

The fibrin monomere interacts with the patient's own factor VIII and calcium to convert the final product into a fibrin polymer that allows for platelets activation and aggregation with subsequent hemostasis.

They are presented with a dual chamber syringe that allows for the combination of the thrombin and fibrinogen when the plunger is depressed. They also can be used in spray. Many commercial products are now on the market: Tisseel (Baxter), Evicel formerly called Crosseal (Johnson and Johnson)...Tisseel is now bovine free.

4. Classification of existing products

4.1 Surgical local hemostatic agents with an aspecific effect on the clotting cascade

Hemostatic agents with a natural origin

Are medical devices of Class III, and may be extracted from animals (calf, ox, pig or horse) or plants (wood, cotton, alga, potatoe-starch)

Mecanism of efficacy

Collagen and gelatine induce the platelet aggregation leading to a clot when in contact with blood

Oxidized cellulosis allows absorption of blood. Glycuronic acid diminishes the PH, induces vasoconstriction, and the creation of hematin film, and in vitro shows an bactericid effect.

Alginates release the Ca++ ions , with a platelet activation followed by a fibrinoformation. Alga fibers reinforce the clot structure.

Starch acts like a filter which concentrate the blood cells and the proteins such as thrombin, albumin and fibrinogen, with an hemostasis occurring in a few minutes.

Different products

Composition	origin	product	presentation
Collagen	Calf	Pangen	compress
	Ox	Avitene	
	Pig	Surgicol	
	Horse	Antema (Biomet)	
		Tissufleece (Baxter) Gentafleece (Baxter) Septocoll (Biomet) + gentamycin Collatemp (Inocoll)	
Gelatin	Ox	Floseal (Baxter) + Thrombin Gelitaspon (Caps recherche)	Gel powder, gel, pad
	Pig	Surgiflo Johnson & Johnson)	gel
		Spongostan (Johnson & Johnson) Gelita (Pouret)	Powder Plugs
Oxidized cellulosis	Wood	Surgicel (Johnson&Johnson)	Compress
	Cotton	Gelitacel (Caps recherché)	
Alginates	Laminaria Hyperborea	Algosterile	Compress
Starch	Potatoe	Arista (Medafor)	Powder

Hemostatic agents with a synthetic origin

Their classification depends on their chemical category

- Aldehyds associated with gelatine (GRF) or albumin (Bioglue –Gamida-)
- Glycol polyethylens (Coseal –Baxter- and pleuraseal)
- Cyanoacrylates (Glubran and Omnex)

Mechanism of efficacy

Their aim is the constitution of a film to obtain water tightness and prevent the risk of hemorrage

They won't be developed here their use being contraindicated in neurosurgery.

4.2 Hemostatic agents with a specific effect on hemostasis cascade

Concern four products containing all fibrinogen and thrombin, their difference is due to the different associated coagulating factors leading to product the last stage of the coagulation (Silver, Wang & AL 1995, Jackson 2001). Experimental studies have compared the properties and efficacy of the different fibrin sealants (Dickneite, Metzner & Al 2003) in correlation with their components. They emphasized the necessity of Factor XIII as the key of a good efficacy for clotting. All tested fibrin sealants performed well on individual parameters, but Beriplast (Aventis Behring) was the foremost fibrin sealant in consistently providing early hemostasis.

These products are the Tissucol, the Beriplast, the Quixil and the Tachosyl.

Each one contains other coagulation factors (Factor XIII, fibronectin,plasminogen), and an antifibrinolytic.

The Quixil contains no substance from animal origin, but transnenamic acid and subsequently must never be in contact with nervous tissues.

Tissucol (Baxter)

- Can exist as a solution or a spray
- *Powder and reconstitution solution I
- Contains human components: fibrinogen (90mg/ml), Factor XIII(10UI/ml), fibronectin(5,5mg/ml), plasminogen0,08mg/ml), bovine aprotinin (3000 UIK/ml)
- *Powder and reconstitution solution II
- Contains human thrombin (500 UI/ml)
- *The excipient of powder and reconstitution I
- Contains glycin, human albumin, sodium nitrate, tyloxapol
- *The excipient of powder and reconstitution solution IIContains Glycin, Sodium chlorure, reconstitution solution EPPI, Calcium chlorure
- Must be kept in refrigerator, can be kept for 2 years
- After reconstitution remains stable for 4 hours

Beriplast (Nycomed)

- Same presentation
- *Powder and reconstitution solution I

- Contains human components: Fibrinogen (90mg/ml), Factor XIII(60UI/ml), with bovine aprotinin (1000UIK/ml)
- *Powder and reconstitution II
- Contains human thrombin (500UI/ml)
- *Powder and reconstitution solution
- Contains human thrombin (500UI/ml)
- *Powder and reconstitution solution I
- Contains Isoleucin, Arginin, Sodium glutamate, human albumin, Sodium citrate, reconstitution EPPI, Sodium chlorure
- Can be kept for one year at room temperature, and 2 in refrigerateur
- Remains stable for 24 hours after preparation.

Quixil (Johnson &Johnson)

We don't detail its composition for the previously related reason.

Tachosil (Nycomed)

Presents as compress

- *The white side is covered with human fibrinogen(5,5mg/cm2
- * The yellow side with human thrombin (2UI/cm2
- The excipients associate horse collagen, human albumin, Riboflavin, sodium chlorure, sodium citrate, L-Arginin.
- Can be kept for three years at room temperature

Autolog fibrin:Vivostat system (Vivolution)

- Is a medical device whose the European autorisation has been given in 2000.
- This automatized system can provide autolog from the patient blood in 23 minutes.
- It associates a processor, a Kit preparation and a spray system.
- It contains no animal component so it eliminates all risks of viral transmission
- Nowadays, it is mainly used in cardiac and thoracic surgery, in vascular and abdominal surgery, but not in neurosurgery.

5. Patches and pads

Those non-invasive hemostatic closure devices as described by Hirsch, Reddy & Al 2003 are mainly used to obtain hemostasis of percutaneous arteriotomy sites of arterial catheterization. This type of patch comes from the studies confirming the hemostatic properties of a high-molecular –weight polysaccharide the poly-N-acetyl-glucosamine (p-Glc-Nac).

Its use is mostly in cardiac surgery and and in interventional radiology.

5.1 Choice of the device and indications

First we shall remind that some specialities are contra-indicated in neurosurgery: cyanoacrylates, Quixil, alginates. H2O2 must only be used out of the dura mater.

The choice of the product and the strategy for local hemostasis are correlated with the type of neurosurgery, the sources of the bleeding, and the neurosurgeon practice, and the financial supplies.

No one must expect from local hemostatic products whatever their quality to be a substitute for the classical bipolar electrocoagulation hemostasis, and more widely for the respect of the tissues.

5.1.1 Type of bleeding

Arterial bleeding

Bipolar coagulation must be used and gives a perfect adequacy to the needs if associated with irrigation.

Bleeding from a venous sinus

The suture remains the best mean when possible, possibly reinforced with a muscle or aponevrotic patch. If the bleeding is close to the vault, the suspension of the dura mater to the bone with interposition of a patch of muscle, oxidized cellulosis or both is the solution.

Anterior cavernous sinus bleeding can be controlled by injection of fibrin glue with a good hemostasis. However of the series reported by Sekhar, Natarajan & Al 2007, of the 20 patients who had an injection in the superior petrosal sinus, 2 experienced complications caused by occlusion of veins draining the brainstem. The 46 whose anterior cavernous sinus had been injected had no complications.

Diffuse bleeding "cloth-bleeding"

A global hemostasis disturbance must be searched.

Local hemostatic agents are indicated, the most often oxidized cellulosis (surgical) will be applied, as well as tissucol (solution or spray).

Bone bleeding

Bone wax remains the most commonly used device, with a good efficacy. However, large amounts must be avoided for they will stay there for ever as a foreing body, and may be the cause of chronic infection, and a secondary removal.

When skull base surgery is performed, surgical, muscle can be on the bleeding site. According to the concerned neurosugeons, the most effective product is the Floseal (powder).

Dura mater water-proof

Prevention of cerebro-spinal fluid (CSF) leaks must be done by the tight closure of the dura mater, reinforced if necessary by application of Surgicel.

Large defects require a graft which can also be sutured, the suture of which may be reinforced in the same way.

In large defects of the dura mater or on the skull base, most of the neurosurgeons will fill the defect with autolog fat tissue (easily indentified on post-operative CT-scan or MRI pictures) associated with glue (Tissucol or Bioglue). An external lumbar CSF derivation will be added in the most difficult cases.

N-B: A local hemostatic agent will never by itself be sufficient to give a definitive water-proof security.

5.2 Main uses in daily practical practice

Skull and brain injuries

The surgery of the skull base defects requires in most of the cases the filling of bone defects with tailed bone grafts, followed by the suture and/or grafting of the dura mater and as previously described the application of a local agent, Surgicel being the most widely used.

Brain contusions require after excision of the necrotic tissues to apply some Surgicel if any small bleeding goes on, the best option being to obtain a very good hemostasis with nothing left in the remaining cavity.

Opened cranio-cerebral wounds must be cleaned with a non-aggressive product, and H2O2 is still indicated in such circumstances.

Transphenoidal surgery

Bleeding during pituitary surgery with a transphenoidal approach can lessen visibility, and this confined narrow route does not allow the use of electrocoagulation. The use of oxidized cellulose or glue is very useful. Ellgala, Maartens & Al 2002 have tested the use Floseal during 293 with a satisfying result.

Endoscopic surgery

The endoscopic treatment of CSF leaks of the anterior skull base whatever their a aetiology, includes the identification of the defect, the filling of the defect with a fragment of the medial turbinate fixed with bioglue followed by appliance of the rest of the pedicled turbinate below and oxidized cellulose (Surgicel) packing.

Same procedures using muscle or turbinate may be used if a leak occurs during an hypophysis surgery procedure, Surgicel being commonly used to maintain the devices and / or to reinforce hemostasis.

Some devices such as catheters are very useful in those deep tight fields.

Spine and spinal cord surgery

Vertebral plexus are better controlled with local hemostatic agents. Fibrin glue is effective when the more common appliance of Surgicel is not effective (Sekhar, Natarajan & Al 2007)

Spinal cord tumors must be approached through laminotomy, the lamina section being done with a craniotomy. After retraction of the posterior arch flap, the extradural hemostasis must be perfect sometimes difficult due to epidural veins. Bipolar coagulation of the veins will be completed by appliance of small fragments of Surgicel, and bone wax on bone section the opening of the spinal cord is done under magnification. Surgicel application will help for hemostasis, the coagulation use being as restricted as possible.

After the tumour removal, no hemostatic agent should be left intradurally. The closing of the dura mater is seldom absolutely waterproof, and Surgicel and glue are commonly used to improve its quality (Lapierre 2009).

In other intra-dural spinal surgery one must avoid to let in situ any agent.

Brain surgery

From the extra-dural stage to the ending of the extradural hemostasis after the dura mater closure, local hemostatic agents have their place all along the procedure, to protect the brain, and to complete local hemostasis (Federspiel, Josephson &Al). In brain tumours, oxidized cellulose (surgical) is widely used, during the ablation of the tumour and at the end of the procedure to prevent and stop any bleeding in the remaining cavity whatever the type of tumor. One must be aware that it is still illegal to let products like Surgicel inside brain cavities, and inside the dura mater. Many physicians however will not take this in account considering the appliance of local agents on previously bleeding walls a better security for the patient. Tschan & Al 2010 have also evaluated the efficacy and safety of micropolysaccaride hemispheres (MPH) with no reported adverse effect. As soon as postoperative day 1, MPH were not detected anymore. There was no tumor mimicking enhancement. Many publications and everyone experience however report signal anomalies on post operative imagery mimicking residual tumour or early recurrence, or even an abcess, or a cotton pad when using Surgicel or gelatine sponge (Maurer, Ekholm & Al 1986)...This has led to some iterative unuseful surgery and even legacy. The histologic study only shows granuloma.

In aneurisms surgery, before the development of interventional radiology, aneurisms who could not be clipped were wrapped with muscle and hemostatic agents, unsuccessfully. Nowadays, surgery of aneurisms only requires hemostatic agents during the procedure to protect the brain and stop the faint bleedins coming from the neighbouring. Appliance of some small Surgicel pieces to the aneurism neck and clip may help to maintain the clip parallel to the vessel direction when releasing the retractors.

Spinal surgery

Local hemostatic agents have many indications in spinal surgery of all types, especially to ensure the epidural veins hemostasis.

They must not be left in contact with nerve roots intra or extradurally, due to the possibility of granuloma formation. Their presence is credited of the appearance of post-operative pain.

In case of epidural spontaneous hematomas they are very useful particularly if they are due to anti-coagulant accidents.

A randomized study performed in 127 patients by Renkens, Payner & Al 2001 comparing Floseal, microfibrillar collagen (Aviten) and fibrin glue showed the control of hemostasis in ten minutes for 97% of the cases with Floseal, and for 71% with the other agents.

6. Listing of main complications

Stroke

Is only reported when using hydrogen peroxide (H_2O_2). Mut, Yemisci & al 2009 reported one case in a patient, after which they performed an experimental study on mice brains using 3% H_2O_2 solution. When H_2O_2 was applied on the cortex, a vasoconstrictive response of all arteries and arterioles of the treated zone was observed, and after 15 seconds of exposure to H_2O_2, multiple bubbles were observed within the lumen of all subpial arteries when pial layer had been destroyed, or not.

Histology revealed the production of peroxynitrite, and the diffusion of H2O2 through the superficial cortical layers. The addition of peroxide and H2O2 resulted in platelet aggregation and acute thrombus formation. The combination of NO and H2O2 is cytotoxic, and mediated by generated NO radicals. Among them, peroxinitrite is a potent and destructive oxdant, which may disrupt the blood-brain barrier.

Those data confirm that H2O2 must only be used in the extra-dural space.

Peripheral nerve impairment

The potential effect of hemostatic agents of peripheral nerve function was suspected by clinical experience of postoperative local deficit or pain after the appliance of hemostatic agents in situ.

Experimental studies heve been performed by Nagamatsu, Podratz & al 1996 and Alkan, Inat & al 2007.

The first used oxicel (OC) (Deseret medical, Becton Dickinson and Company, Sandy, Utah) for studies in vitro and in vivo in rats. In vitro, neurite outgrowth of the dorsal root ganglion neuron was inhibited after 15 minutes exposure

In vivo, the Ph was lowered in the subperineurium, and remained low for 2 hours. The acidity of the oxidised cellulose is involved in the development of experimental neuropathy by OC. The direct application of OC to peripheral nerves must be avoided.

The second studied the effect of oxidized regenerated cellulose, gelatine sponge, bone wax and bovine collagen on the sciatic nerve of the rat, embedded in each substance. The compound action potential (CAP), and the nerve conduction velocity (NCV) were studied one hour and four weeks after the operation. In the bovine collagen and bone wax groups they were no statistically significant differences compared with initial control group.

In the gelatine sponge group, CAP was increased statistically significantly 4 weeks after surgery.

In the oxidized regenerated cellulose, NCV was significantly reduced, and the CAP increased 1 hour after surgery. No significant difference was seen after 4 weeks, but partial necrosis and walking disturbances were seen on the operated legs after 1 to 3 weeks.

Bovine collagen seems the most adapted for direct appliance to the nerves.

Intra-spinal retained Surgicel can induce radiculopathy (Partheni, Kalogheropouplou & Al 2006) and MRI studies could not exclude a post-operative hematoma, leading to reoperate the patient

Granulomatous formations

When left in the operative field, hemostatic agents may induce early or late tissue reactions and the formation of granulomas especially oxidized cellulose (Voormolen, Ringers & Al 1987) . Kaymaz, Tokgoz & al 2005, in an experimental study in the rabbit brain report the modifications due to the application of oxidized cellulose and gelatine sponge. They observe on MRI a perilesional oedema in both series, while histopathology a tissue-degeneration more marked with the gelatine sponge use 24 hours after operation. In a rat brain neurosurgical model (228 animals), Ereth, Schaff & Al 2008 studied Arista, Surgicel, Avitene,

Floseal or Kaolin (positive control) and showed the presence of residual material in all animals with Avitene, Surgicel and Floseal at day 14. Avitene and Floseal demonstrated a propensy for causing granuloma formation.

Apel-Sarid, Cochrane &Al 2010 report a pediatric case series of 3 patients: the 3 cases had intra cerebral surgery (2 for tumors ablations, and one focal dysplasy treatment). The local hemostatic used agent was microfibrillar collagen haemostat (Avitene). The three had a second surgery for new or recurrent seizures, and MRI exploration suspected either a tumour recurrence or an abscess. Histologically, the mixed inflammatory infiltrate was typified by the presence of Avitene-centric necrotizing granulomas surrounded by a palisade of macrophages and often several eosinophils.

So long, one must remain aware that the best behaviour is to remove any local hemostatic agent before closing the dura, if possible.

Viral transmission

With purified products, the risk of viral transmission has become very weak but is not totally missing, since all the products contain bovine components except for Vivostat. No recent report has been published yet. Virally inactivated human thrombin has replaced now bovine thrombin in most European products. (Buttusil 2003)

Antibodies formation and immunologic concerns

In the series of Renkens, Payner & Al 2001, at 6-8 weeks post operative evaluation of antibodies again bovine thrombin and bovine FactorVa demonstrated no stastical significance in the differences between treatment and control groups.

There was no evidence of antibody-related coagulopathy in either group. However, immunology mediated coagulopathy associated with exposure to bovine thromin or to fibrin sealants containing this component is widely recognized. This component had to be replaced by human thrombin (Buttusil 2003). Bovine aprotinin (BA) may induce severe anaphylactic reactions, especially in patients previously treated with such products, suggesting that the use of a test dose should be proposed.

Crosseal A containing traneximic acid (TA) eliminates this risk, but is contraindicated for neurosurgery.

7. Financial point of view for hemostatic agents

The most sophisticated they are, the most expansive. Anyway, the most daily used of all remain the oxidized cellulose, and the coast remains important. I should dare to add considering the glues that during the 15 years of my practice they did not exist. When they were available I have been using them for the ten following years.

After some warning about security, I stopped. The results remain identical during these three consecutive periods.

In developing countries, the price remains prohibitive, and in other countries, the local hemostatic agents are probably widely over-used. The indispensable devices remain electrocoagulation, Horsley wax, associated with a cautious and accurate surgery. The indication of local hemostatic agents must be evaluated in terms of rik-benefit for the patient, and not considered as a comfort for the surgeon. Of course local hemostatic agents are useful in some cases, but must not considered as compulsory in the daily practice.

8. Disclosure

The authors report no conflict of interest concerning the materials ad devices described in this paper.

9. References

Abaut, A-Y, Basle, B. 2008, Les agents hémostatiques chirurgicaux, *Pharm Hosp* 43, 2-8

Alkan, A, Inal, S, Yildirim, M, Bas, b, Agar, E. 2007. The effects of hemostatic agents on peripheral nerve function: An experimental study. *J oral maxillofac Surg* 65, 6306-634

Apel-sarid, L, Cochrane, D, D, Steinbok, P, Byrne, A, T, Dunham, C.2010. Microfibrillar collagen haemostat-induced necrotizing granulomatous inflammation developing after craniotomy: a pediatric case series. *J Neurosurg Pediatrics* 6, 385-392

Busuttil, R, W. 2003. A comparison of antifirinolytic agents used in hemostatic fibrin sealants. *J Am Coll Surg*, 197, 6 , 1021-1028

Dickneite, G, Metzner, H, Pfeifer, T, Kroez, M, Witzke, G. 2003. A comparison of fibrin sealants in relation to their in vitro and in vivo properties. *Thrombosis research* 112, 73-82

Dona, C, Vaccino.C. 2009. Topical hemostasis: a valuable adjunct to control bleeding in the operating room, with a special focus on thrombinand fibrin sealants. *Informa Phamaceutical Science* 2. 243-247

Ellegala, D, B, Maartens, N, F, Laws, E, R. 2001. Use of floseal hemostatic sealant in transphenoidal pituitary surgery: Technical note. *Neurosurgery* 51, 513-516

Ereth-Mark, H, Schaft, M, Ericson, E, Wetgen, N, Nuttal, G, Oliver, W, C, 2008. Comparative safety and efficacy of topical hemostatic agents in a rat neurosurgical model. *Neurosurgery*, 63, 369-372

Federspiel, F, Josephson, A, Dardelle, D, Gaillard, S, Letailleur, M. 2008. Utilisation des agents hémostatiques en neurochirurgie. *Pharm Hosp* 43, 9-13

Fincher, E, 1946. Further uses of gelatine foam in neurosurgeryPresented at the meeting of the Harvey Cushing Society, October 12, Boston MasschussettsHarvey *Cushing Society Reports* 97-104

Grant, G. 2007. Update on hemostasis: neurosurgery. *SurgeryS55*, 142, 4S, S55-S60

Hawiger, j. 1987. Formation and regulation of platelet and fibrin hemostatic Plug. *Human pathology* 18, 2, 111-122

Hirsch, J, A, Reddy, S, A, Capasso, W, E, Linfante, I. 2003. Non-invasive hemostatic closure devices: "Patches and Pads". *Techniques in Vascular and Interventional Radiology*, 6, 2, 92-95

Ito, H, Onishi, H, Shoin, K, Nagatani, H. 1989. Granuloma caused by oxidized cellulose following craniotomy. *Acta Neurochirurgica*, 100, 1-2

Jackson, M, R. 2001. Fibrin sealants in surgical practice: an overview. *The American Journal of surgery* 182 1S-7S

Kaymaz, m, Tokgoz, N, Kardes, O, Özköse, z, Özogui, c, Orbay, t. 2005. Radiological and histopathological examination of early tissue reactions to absorbable hemostatic agents in the rabbit brain. *Journal of clinical neuroscience.* 12, 4, 445-448

Kothbauer, K, R, Jallo, G, I, Siffert, J, Jimenez, E, Allen, J, C, Epstein, F, J. 2001. Foreing body reaction to hemostasis materials mimicking recurrent brain tumor. *J Neurosurg*, 95, 0503

Krause, D.2008. Regulatory history of adsorbable hemostatic agents and dressings. *Le pharmacien hospitalier(hors série1)*, 84, 3716

Lapierre, F. 2009. Les agents hémostatiques locaux en neurochirurgie: note technique. *Neurochirurgie*, 55 Hors série 1, 40-44

Light Upjohn Richard 1945. Hemostasis in neurosurgery Harvey *Cushing Society Reports* 414-434

Maurer, P, K, Ekholm, S, E, Mac Donald, J, V, Sands, M, Kido, D. 1986. Postoperative radiographic appearance of intracranial hemostatic gelatine sponge. *Surgical Neurology* 26, -, 562-566

Mut, M, Yemisi, m, Gursov-Ozdemir, Y, Ture, U. 2009. Hydrogen peroxide induced stroke: elucidation of the mechanism in vivo. *J Neurosurg* 110, 94-100

Nagamatsu, M, Podratz, j, Windebank, A, J, Low, P, A. 1997, Acidity is involved in the development of neuropathy caused by oxidized cellulose. *Journal of the neurological sciences* 146, 97-102

Partheni, m, lalogheropoulou, C, Karageorgos, N, Paniagiotopoulos, V, Voulgaris, S, Tzortzidis, F. 2006. Radiculopathy after lumbar discectomy due to intraspinal retained surgical: clinical and magnetic resonance imaging evaluation. *The spine Journal* 6, 455- 458

Peng, C, W, Chou, B, T, Bendo, J, A. 2009. Vertebral artery injury in cervical spine surgery: anatomical considerations, management and preventive measures. *The spine Journal*, 9, 70-76.

Renchengary, S, S. 1993 . Principles of neurosurgery. Wilkins R.H, 1;18-19

Renkens, K, L Jr, Payner, T, D, Leipzig, T, J, Feuer, H, Morone, M, A, Koers, J, M, Lawson, K, J, Lentz, R, Shuey, H Jr, Conaway, G, L, Andersson, G, B, An, A, S, Hickey, m, Rondinone, J, F, Shargill, N, S. 2001. A multicenter, prospective, randomized trial evaluating a new agent for spinal surgery. *Spine* , 26, 1645-1650

Rousou, J, Levitsky, S, Gonzalez-Lavin, L, Cosgrove, D, Magilligan, D, Weldon, C, Hiebert, c, Hess, P, Joyce, L, Bergsland, J. 1989? Randomized clinical trial of fibrin sealant in patients undergoing resternotomy or reinterventional cardiac operations: a multicenter study. *J Thoracic Cardiovasc surgery* , 97, 687-693

Satkunurath, K, Royston, D, 2008. Hemostatic drugs in trauma and orthopaedic practice. *Traumacare*, 1, 24-29

, D, 2007.The use of fibrin glue to stop venous bleeding in the epidural space, vertebral venous plexus, and anterior cavernous sinus: technical note. *Operative neurosurgery* I, 61,

Seyednejad, H, Imani, M, Jamieson, T, Seifalian, A, M. 2008. Topical hemostatic agents. *Br J Surg* 95, 1195-1225

Spiller, M, Tenner, M, S, Couldwell, W, T. 2001. Effect of absorbable hemostatic agents on the relaxation time blood: An in vitro study with implications for post-operative MRI. *J neurosurg* 95, 687-693

Silver, F, H, Wang M-C, Pins, G, D, 1995. Preparation and use of fibrin glue in surgery. *Biomaterials* 16, 891-903

Tschan, W, T, 2010, Rahmen Der Neurowoche, GMS Publishing House, Doc P 1740. http//creative commons, org/licenced/by-nc-nd/30/deed.de-

Voormolen, J, H, C, Ringers, J, Bots, G, A, M, Van Der Heide, A, Hermans, J. 1987. Hemostatic agents: Brain tissue reaction and effectiveness. *Neurosurgery* 20, 5, 702-709

10

Use of Physical Restraints in Neurosurgery: Guide for a Good Practice

Ayten Demir Zencirci
Ankara University, Faculty of Health Sciences, Nursing Department
Turkey

1. Introduction

Physical restraints are widely used in hospitals in many countries, especially during critical care, against a range of difficult clinical situations. They are intended to protect patients and their relatives from any harm to themselves: falling from beds, removing tubes, drains, and medical equipments from their bodies, and to ease patients' control (Bower & McCullough, 2000).

Weaning from artificial ventilation, recovering from acute illness can be a long and difficult process. The problem with critically ill patients is re-sedation, often needed to handle agitation and avoid treatment interference (Cohen et al., 2002). Sedatives lengthen hospitalization and complicate recovery (Westcott, 1995); therefore, the management of these patients can often be a dilemma (Hine, 2007).

1.1 What is a restraint?

Physical restraint is (American Nurses Assosication, 2001) "any chemical or physical involuntary method restricting an individual's movement, physical activity, or normal access to the body."

Physical restraint is also defined as any device, material, or equipment attached to or near a person's body, neither controlled nor easily removed by a patient and that deliberately prevents or intended to prevent free body movement to a position of choice or patients normal access to their body (Retsas, 1998).

1.2 History of physical restraint

Physical restraint use in acute and intensive cares dates back long. While actions –against restraint were taken in England and France during the 19th century, its use in acute care settings in the US was assumed as a therapeutic and morally correct approach against accidents and injures (Bower & McCullough, 2000). In the 1980s, physical restraint applications in acute care settings were on general medical-surgical units (Frengley & Mion, 1986; Lofgren et al., 1989; Mion et al., 1989; Robbins et al., 1987).

Restraint use has become a legal issue with individual rights becoming paramount in the society. First in the USA, federal restraint standards were implemented in 1984 (U.S.

Department of Health and Human Services, 1984). The Mental Health Act of 1983, Wales, (Department of Health and Welsh Office, 1999) named five common reasons to use the restraint, of which three were the most relevant in critical care settings: noncompliance with treatment, self-harm, and risk of a physical injury by an accident. Canada and British Columbia have legislations (Currie, 1997). While the UK, however, does not accept physical restraint use at all, it is common in the US, Australia, and Europe (Maccioli et al., 2003; Royal College of Nursing, 2004; Van Norman & Palmer, 2001). Nurses and scientists from other disciplines tried to agree on physical restraint use starting in 1988 no consensus reached yet on its use in hospitals (Bower & McCullough, 2000).

2. Alternative procedures

Other strategies to manage agitation include :

- Sedation: agitation is often managed with the use of sedatives or antipsychotic drugs ; however, drugs could ultimately lead to further agitation and a vicious circle ensues. The overuse of sedatives could also complicate a patient's recovery by causing hypotension and apnea and by exposing the patient to risks associated with immobility (Westcott, 1995; Woodrow, 2000).
- Communication with patients, relatives
- Touch
- Involvement of family
- Massage
- Acupuncture (Bray et al., 2004)

2.1 Barriers hindering restraint elimination

Research has clearly established that physical restraints can be injurious both physically and mentally for inhabitants, cost more resources, and increase serious injuries.

Barriers to shortening the restraint use included: fear of patient injury, staff and resource restrictions, lack of education and information about alternatives to restraints, policy and management issues, beliefs and expectations (of staff, family and residents), inadequate review practices and statement barriers (Moore & Haralambous 2007).

Perceived barriers to individualized care identified were insufficient staff, safety and authoritarian concerns, lack of team collaboration and phone call, lack of participation by the nursing assistants for care planning, and staff and family attitudes (Walker et al., 1999).

Staff or family attitudes and fears can stop success with restraint elimination measures. The restraint team should be practical and provide education and resources, permit individuals to express their fears and suspicions, and encourage active involvement in designing the plan of care. Approaching restraint decline with an incremental plan allows caregivers to conquer their fears and resistance. Beginning with one unit at a time or starting with the easiest residents and working toward the more difficult may make the task of restraint reduction more reasonable (Castle & Mor, 1998). The successful interventions will allow staff and family members to become more relaxed and convinced with the removal of restraints.

3. Indications and contraindications

Physical restraints are indicated for patient safety and avoiding falls, but the most widespread reason is to put off the taking away of invasive tubes and devices (Fletcher, 1996; Cruz et al., 1997; Minnick et al., 1998; Happ, 2000; Choi and Song 2003). Patients might need repeatedly to be self-extubated while patients was physically restrained (Balon 2001) and restrained patients of self-extubation rate were 77% (Birkett et al, 2005) .

Delirium and agitation been the most frequent hospital complications in 'older' patients, resulting in poor hospital outcomes and increased morbidity and death (Ely et al., 2001), physical restraints are frequently used in this setting, ranging in the literature between 8-68% for hospitalized elderly people (Hamers & Huizing 2005).

3.1 The use of physical restraint in critical care

The intensive care environment itself may grow added stress and agitation, caused by mechanical ventilation, invasive procedures, pain, fear, anxiety, sensory overload and sleep cycle disruptions (Haskell et al., 1997). Incidence of agitation rose because of higher number of of older and more severely ill patients in intensive care units (ICU) (Cohen et al., 2002). However, the prevalence of agitation and delirium in ICU varied between 15 - 87% of patients (Sanders et al., 1992; Ely et al., 2001; Roberts, 2001). This variation could be due to numerous factors and definitions utilized to describe altered mental status: delirium, acute confusional state, sundown syndrome, ICU psychosis and ICU delirium (Haskell et al., 1997).

Agitated patients exhibits constant fidgeting and movement; pulling at bed sheets, invasive devices and catheters; trying to get out of bed; shouting and hitting and were disorientated to the time and the place (Haskell et al., 1997; Cohen et al., 2002). The agitations in critically ill adults are associated with potentially dangerous complications: self-extubation (self-removal of endotracheal tube), removal of arterial and venous lines and non-compliance with life-saving treatment (Cohen et al., 2002; Nirmalan et al., 2004). Ultimately, the presence of agitation delayed weaning from ventilation and lengthened ICU stay (Westcott, 1995; haskell et al., 1997; Cull & Inwood, 1999; Cohen et al., 2002).

Systematically reviewed physical restraint use ranged 3.4- 21% in acute care patients, who were physically restrained for 2.7 to 4.5 days during their hospitalization. The range in residential care settings was between 12%, 47%, and 32%, respectively. The restraint applied was 20 days at least in each month (Evans et al., 2002). Patients were restrained at 6-13%, with higher rates (18- 22%) as well for people 65 years or older. The most common reason for physical restraint was to prevent falls (up to 77%) and disruption of therapy (up to 40%) (MacPherson et al., 1990; Mion et al., 1989). Rates varied in different countries: less than 9% in Denmark, Iceland, and Japan; between 15- 17% in France, Italy, Sweden, and the US, the highest use, almost 40% in Spain (Ljunggren et al., 1997).

However, physical restraint is contraindicated edema and cyanosis, pressure ulcers, aspiration and breathing problems, agitation, contractures, fractures, paralyz and most importantly if the informed consent is not obtained from patients or surrogates (Demir, 2007a; Demir, 2007b).

4. Key step of the procedure

4.1 Types of physical restraints

There are a number of kinds of restraints. The most common restraint devices are wrist restraints (Minnick et al., 1998, Happ, 2000), ankle restraint (Demir, 2007a) and chest or waist restraints (Carrion et al., 2000; Demir, 2007a). Boxing gloves or mittens, involved wrapping the hands in bandages to prevent free use of the fingers (Fletcher, 1996; Nirmalan et al., 2004), therefore preventing the patient from grabbing and pulling at tubes and lines (Demir, 2007a), are also popular. Among the most frequent for adults are jacket restraints, belt restraints, mit for hand restraints, and limb restraints. Restraints for infants and children include mummy restraints, elbow restraints and crib nets (Kozier et al., 2004).

Jacket (body restraint): A sleeveless vest with straps that cross in front or back of the patient and are tied to the bed edge or chair legs.

Belt: Straps or belts applied transversely the patient to save him or her to the stretcher, bed, or wheelchair.

Mitten or hand: Enclosed cloth fabric applied over the patient's hand to put off injury from scratching

Elbow: A combination of cloth and plastic or wooden tongue blades that halt the elbow to prevent flexion.

Limb or extremity: Cloth devices that stop one or all limbs by firmly tying the restraint to the bed frame or chair.

Mummy: A blanket or sheet that is folded around the child to bound the movement. Mummy restraints are used to execute procedures on children.

4.2 General principles for the care of restrained patients

- The purpose of restraint is to provide optimal care of the patient,
- Use of restraint must not be an alternative to insufficient human or other resources
- Restraint should only be used when alternative therapeutic measures have seemed ineffective to acquire the desired outcome,
- Decisions regarding use or non-use of after a detailed patient assessment, by an interdisciplinary team,
- Critical care areas must develop and implement protocol/guidelines in order to aid nurses and others,
- Whatever form of restraint is used there must be suitable, continual evaluation tools used and the findings acted upon,
- Clear, concise documentation of decisions, plans and treatment must be kept within the patients' record,
- The patient and their family should be engaged within discussions to inform them of the reason for choice of the restraint method,
- Schooling all staff regarding chemical, physical and psychological restraint must take in training and competency programs in critical care units (BACCN position in Bray et al., 2004).

4.3 Application guidelines

- Obtain consent from the patient and surrogate,
- Enlighten rationale for application of restraint,
- Select the appropriate type of restraint,
- Assess skin for discomfor,
- Apply restraint to patient assuring some movement of body part. One to two fingers should slide between restraint and patient's skin. Tie straps securely with clove hitch knot,
- Lock restraint to bed frame; do not tie the straps to the side rail,
- Assess restraints and skin integrity every 30 minutes,
- Discharge restraints at least every 2 hours,
- Continually appraise the need for restraints (at least every 4-8 hours),
- Guarantee that a physician's order has been provided or, in an emergency, obtain one within 24 hours after applying the restraint,
- Assure the patient and the patient's people that the restraint is impermanent and protective,
- Apply the restraint in a way that the patients can move as freely as possible without defeating the idea of the restraint,
- Ensure that limb restraints are applied securely but not so tightly that they obstruct blood flow to anybody area or extremity,
- Pad bony prominence (e.g., wrist and ankles) before applying a restraint over them. The movements of a restraint without stuffing over such prominences can quickly erode the skin,
- Constantly tie a limb restraint with a knot (e.g., a clove hitch) that will not tighten when pulled,
- Tie the ends of a body restraint to the part of the bed that moves to lift the head. Never tie the ends to a side rail or to the set frame of the bed if the bed position is to be altered,
- Asses the restraint every 30 minutes. Some services have specific forms to be used to document ongoing assessment,
- Free all restraints at least every 2 to 4 hours, and provide range-of-motion train and skin care,
- Reassess the continued requirement for the restraint at least every 8 hours. Embrace an assessment of the fundamental source of the behavior necessitating use of the restraints,
- When a restraint is momentarily removed, do not leave the client alone,
- Instantly report to the nurse in charge and record on the client's chart any constant reddened or broken skin areas under the restraint,
- At the first sign of cyanosis or pallor, coldness of a skin area, or a client's complaint of a tingling feeling, pain, or numbness, release the restraint and exercise the limb,
- Apply a restraint so that it can be freed quickly in an emergency and with the body part in a typical anatomic position,
- Offer emotional support verbally and through touch (Kozier et al., 2004, Taylor et al., 1997).

4.4 JCAHO restraint standards for non-psychiatric patients

Special Conditions When Restraint Is Applied:

- Based on important alteration in the patient's state with the physician notified immediately and written orders obtained within 24 hours

- Initiated by a registered nurse
- Based on protocols customary for situations where patients may hurt themselves if staff initiate, maintain, and terminate restraint without an order from autonomous practitioner

Organizational Perspective:

- Be specific for each institution
- Exhibit clinical justification
- Exhibit the use of innovative alternatives
- Outline preventive strategies
- Name ways to reduce risks associated with restraint use

Policies/Procedures/Protocols:

- Be clearly declared
- Advocate use of least limiting measures

Preventive Strategies:

- Identify potentially risky patient behaviors
- Identify efficient and tried alternatives

Plan of Care

- Individualized and guarantee patient's assessed needs are met
- Conserve patient's rights, dignity, and well-being

Education:

- Be continuing for staff and patient
- Be provided to families when fitting

Initiation and Monitoring of Restraint Use:

- Based on state law
- Initiated based on individual orders or approved
- Protocols with written physician order obtained within 12 hours
- Applied/monitored/assessed/reassessed by qualified staff
- Monitored at least every 2 hours
- Obtained a new permission for every 24 hours when continuous restraint is used

Documentation:

- Incorporate all restraint episodes according to organizational policies and procedures
- Record , at a minimum, every 2 hours
- Specify alternatives tried before restraints were applied
- Write in into the patient's medical record

Key elements of restraint documentation

- Reason for the restraint
- Method of restraint
- Application: Date, time, and patient's response

- Duration
- Frequency of observation and patient's response
- Safety: Release from restraint with periodic, routine exercise and assessment for flow and skin integrity
- Assessment of the continuous demand for restraint
- Patient outcome

5. Complications of physical restraint

Increasing awareness of its negative effects and its limited efficacy in the last decade reduced the use of physical restraint. One hundred deaths in the USA occur annually in addition to higher hospital infection rates and injuries by improper physical restraint. Moreover, patients under physical restraint lost muscle strength, had pressure ulcers, incontinence, strangulation (Taylor et al., 1997), and were severely agitated, confused, depressed, angry, fearful, confused, panicked, and experienced sleeping difficulties, loss of role, shyness, body disformation, resistance or objection to daily routine activities, higher disorganized behaviours, cognitive and behavioural problems due to changes in blood chemistry, and loss of self-trust and respect (Bonner et al., 2002; Bray et al., 2004; Cannon et al., 2001; Castle, 2002; Choi & Song, 2003; Evans et al., 2002, 2003; Hem et al., 2001; Koch & Lyon, 2001; Shorr et al., 2002; Swauger & Tomlin, 2000). Avoiding physical injuries by physical restraint is only possible through improved quality of care. The rules were by the Health Care Financing Administration in 1987 and Joint Commission on Accreditation of Healthcare Organizations (JCAHO; Taylor et al., 1997). Government and accreditation organizations have supported the decisions on physical restraint use in the last 15-20 years because of increased significance of patients' rights.

Over the last 20 years there has been an increasing evidence supporting the reduction of restraints' use of. Some complications reported by Demir (2007a) were: edema and cyanosis by wrist and arm restraints, pressure ulcers, aspiration and breathing problems caused by sheet and belt pressure on chest, head hits by angry patients on bed sides, contractures of joints, and rejecting meals. Nine patients were suffocated when tied up with sheet on the chest, two had humerus fractures, two needed head skin sutures after falling out of bed, and one was paralyzed after being tied to the bed by the arms.

Atrioventricular irregularities in elderly patients on whom limb and vest restrained were observed (Evans et al., 2003). After longer periods of agitation, tachycardia and deaths were experienced. Mott et al. (2005) stated that physical restraint did not fully serve the purpose and increased agitation. Sullivan-Marx and colleagues' (1999) reported a higher risk of falls and strangulation (Lee et al., 1999) as well. Time restrained patients spent in hospitals were longer than unrestrained patients and experienced higher risks of complications, lower discharges from hospitals, and higher death risks (Arbesman & Wright, 1999; Clary & Krishnan, 2001; Paterson et al., 2003).

Asphyxiation, the most common cause of restraint related death, is termed as "restraint asphyxia" in the forensic and emergency literature by Reay (1998). Death occurred in approximately 12% of cases of a total of 214 episodes of hobble tying in agitated delirium (Stratton et al., 2001). There were various reports: 131 deaths to the FDA, USA, from 1987–1996, for the manufacturers of protective restraints (Morrison, 1997) , 58 asphyxia occurrences out of 770 cases and 44 wheel chair related fatal accidents out of 58 cases (Calder & Kirby 1990), also reported. Higher physical restraint with agitation, more complications and frequent fell down (Shorr et al., 2002).

6. Ethical and legal considerations on restraint use

All nurses (/health professionals) have a duty to safeguard and protect their patients from harm. The nurse's moral obligation is to do no harm (non-maleficence) and promote good (beneficence). It might also be conflicting for critical care nurses, when they are to maintain a safe environment for agitated and delirious patients and also the potentially lifesaving technological devices. The picture is even more complex by the nurse's obligation to ensure patient freedom, dignity, and autonomy (Reigle, 1996). Since everyone has the right to be free from forced restraint of movement, torture or degrading treatment (HMSO, 1998), nurses have to justify use of physical restraint (Kapp, 1996). However, the literature contained very little evidence of restraints providing protection. So researchers debates just how ethical are the use of physical restraints.

The nurse's responsibility is to respect patient autonomy, whereas the use of physical restraint violates the principles of informed consent. Since restraint is a non-validated therapy, their use is considered investigational and a higher standard of informed consent should be required (Moss & LaPuma, 1991). Providing informed consent implies that the patient is competent to take the information on board; however, if physical restraint is being considered, the patient is probably agitated and less likely to have the capacity to give informed consent (Royal College of Nursing, 2004). Although the Department of Health (2001) guidelines are clear that no one is able to give consent on behalf of another, communication with the patient and the relatives on the rationale for restraint remains paramount. The reasonable person' rule can be applied in such cases, which enables a professional to act in the best interests of the patient (Beauchamp & Childress, 2001). A reasonable person is the one who would wish to be treated for life-threatening conditions even not able to give consent (Dimond , 2002). When there are other available alternatives, however, health care professionals should not assume that a reasonable person would wish to be physically restrained. Admittedly, the alternatives include other methods of restraint in the form of sedation, which itself can prolong and complicate a patient's recovery.

The Mental Capacity Act (Deparment of Constitutional Affairs, 2005) states that anything done for or on behalf of individuals without capacity, for example restraint, must be the least restrictive of their basic rights and freedoms and be in their best interests. If restraint is to be in the patient's best interest, health care professionals must have been satisfied by all legal and ethical implications, since otherwise they might face allegations of assault (Deparment of Health, 2001). Crucial differences exist between restraint that violates rights and dignity and restraint that does not violate any autonomously expressed wishes protects the patient from self-harm and is in the patients' best interests (Nirmalan et al., 2004). However, the evidences discussed previously, exposing the patient to potential harmful effects from restraint is in their best interests is debatable.

6.1 Informed consent

Consent from patients or surrogates for all healthcare activities and medical treatments are a must since fundamental moral duty forbids any actions against a person's wishes and dignity. Informed consent thus entails a shared decision by both patient and health professional (Andanda, 2005). If a patient has a doubtful capacity, health care professionals have to take necessary steps against deterioration first and then consider capacity and consent matters (English et al., 2004).

Informed consent is widely recognized in international guidelines (Bandman & Bandman, 2002; International Council of Nurses, 2001) and in legislation (Department of Health and Welsh Office, 1999). There are four basic elements of informed consent, developed starting with Nuremberg trials (Andanda, 2005), which are also valid for patient care:

• "Capacity to consent;
• Full disclosure of relevant information;
• Adequate comprehension of the information by the participant;
• Voluntary decision to participate and withdraw from participation at any stage without prejudice of the participant. Participant withdrawal should be accepted and withdrawing participants should not be expected to give any reasons for their decision."

One could evaluate informed consent well only if she has a good understanding of human rights and ethics. Human rights are defined by the American Nurses Association (ANA) as "assertions that call for treating human beings as ends in them, rather than as goals or purposes of others" (Bandman & Bandman, 2002). Ethical principles, of which three guides for all care activity used by nurses are the following: respect for persons, beneficence, and justice. These principles were at the US federal level in the Belmont Report in 1979 (The National Commission for the Protection of Human Subjects of Biomedical and Behavioral Research (NCPHS]) (Burns & Grove, 1999). The dignity and rights of the patient are before the goals of any research or anything since many medical or nursing cares, though acceptable, could be harmful or outweigh the expected benefits (English et al., 2004).

The recent studies on informed and shared decision within clinical care have revealed a pronounced tension among three competing factors:

• Paternalistic conservatism about information exposé to patients has been worn by moral arguments and largely established by the medical profession,
• While many patients may wish to be given information about available treatment options, many also emerge cognitively and psychologically too ill to understand and to hold it, and
• Even when patients do comprehend information about likely treatment options; they do not essentially wish to make such choices themselves and might prefer to leave final decisions to the clinicians.

The second and third factors apparently disagree with the first and make the case more difficult (Doyal, 2001).

Physical restraint has become a common method for difficult clinical situations in hospitals although it has been well recognized in years that nurses should obtain consent from the patient before any nursing care procedure (Bandman & Bandman, 2002; Aveyard, 2005). Similarly, informed consent has become a common method of protecting patients and health care givers as well (Kanerva, 1999) from unexpected cost of physical restraint use, because of increased concern for human and patient rights in the USA and the UK. While physical restraint is required or essential in patients with unsatisfactory mental (Bridgman & Wilson, 2000) or decision-making capacity (Harrison et al., 1997) or psychiatric patients, informed consent is still a must and be, at least, obtained from surrogates (Usher & Arthur, 1998). In other words, a patient at any stage, or under any circumstances is to agree or to disagree with a certain treatment (Beauchamp & Childress, 2001).

Some codes of ethics and regulations are in use in a variety of countries but there are few in Turkey. Only existing code is "Medicine and professional ethics", which was accepted in 1960 and later revised in 1998 (Turkish Medical Association, 1999). The Patients' Rights Regulations placed into effect by the Ministry of Health in August 1998 is the first and only regulation (The General Directorate of Development of Regulations and Publishing, 1998). The content of these is similar to the Declaration on the Promotion of Patients' Rights' in Europe (World Health Organization, 1994). More, however, has to be implemented in Turkey to avoid misguided / misused physical restraint without informed consent and its consequences of legal challenges for maltreatment, negligence, or human rights. However, Demir-Zencirci (2009) stated that most of nurses in her study (97.6%, n= 248) used physical restraint without informed consent.

The aim of informed consent is to protect the autonomous choices of vulnerable persons such as physically restrained patients. Informed consent for medical interventions should be based on size and likelihood of the risks associated with the proposed intervention. As the risks associated with the use of physical restraints are significant, consent for their use is crucial (Reigle, 1997).

7. Illustrative cases

Case 1

A 21 year old male patient was hospitalized in neurosurgery because of a car accident resulted in depressed fracture on left temporal and subarachnoid hemorrhage. Three-four cm laceration existed on right deltoid anterior. When arrived to Emergency Unit via 112, he experienced extensive respiratory distress and higher arterial blood pressure. Ear Nose Throat Department failed to insert endotracheal tubes, therefore, opened tracheostomy. He was unconscious and his orientation and cooperation were not assessed. The patient had extensior on the upper extremity and flexor attracts on the lower extremity via painful stimuli. Vital signs were, later on, normalized. White blood cells were too high (29.200/L), SaO_2 was 94.3%, blood ph was 7.34, Gag reflex was positive, and no neck stiffness. Patient was physically restrained on wrists and ankles.

Aplication

- Provided a physician order.
- Explained to the surrogate what you are going to do, why it is necessary, and how they cooperate.
- Discussed with the surrogate how the results will be used in planning further care or treatments.
- Allowed time for the surrogate to express feelings about being tied/restrained.
- Provided needed emotional reassurance that the restraints will be used only when absolutely necessary and that there will be close contact with the surrogate in case assistance is required.

- Provided a written informed consent from his legal surrogate/his father.
- Washed hands and observed appropriate infection control procedures.
- Provided for patient privacy.
- Applied the wrist and ankle restraint with cotton ties.
- Pad put on bony prominences on the wrist and ankle for to prevent skin abrasion.
- Pulled the tie of the restraint through the slit in the wrist portion or through the buckle.
- Assessed restraints and skin integrity every 30 minutes.
- Discharged restraints at least every 2 hours.
- Appraised the need for restraints for every 4-8 hours.
- Stopped the restraint and applied the exercises on the limb and changed the position for there was cyanosis and pallor, coldness of a skin area.

Mr. A was discharged on foot from neurosurgery intensive care units after 29 days. Physical restraint was applied only 24 days and no complications occurred.

Case 2

A 51 year old female patient with headache, nausea and vomiting got in to the acute care settings. Patient has experienced lethargy and vomiting for three days. She has been brought to the hospital because of increased lethargy. Findings were confusion, lethargic, roughly intact cranial nerves. She reflected no pathologic reflex. Hiperdans parallel with subarachnoid hemorrhage on cranial ct and aneurysmal dilatation on Distal Middle Cerebral Artery were observed. Patient was hospitalized and in neurosurgery intensive care unit and anti-edema and antiepileptic therapy were inititiated.

Confusional, defective orientation and co-operation are observed. Four fifth muscle strength, no pathologic reflex, and (+) neck stiffness. Blood values: Aspartate Aminotransferase (AST) and Gamma Glutamyl Transferase (GGT), Blood urea nitrogen and Creatinine high at range, hemoglobin low at range.

Patient was physically strained on right elbow and ankle.

Aplication

- Provided a physician order.
- Explained to the surrogate what you are going to do, why it is necessary, and how they cooperate.
- Discussed with the surrogate how the results will be used in planning further care or treatments.
- Allowed time for the surrogate to express feelings about being tied/restrained.
- Provided needed emotional reassurance that the restraints will be used only when absolutely necessary and that there will be close contact with the surrogate in case assistance is required.
- Provided a written informed consent from her legal surrogate/her husband.
- Washed hands and observed appropriate infection control procedures.
- Provided for patient privacy.
- Applied the wrist and ankle restraint with cotton ties.
- Pad put on bony prominences on the wrist and ankle for to prevent skin abrasion.
- Pulled the tie of the restraint through the slit in the wrist portion or through the buckle.

- Assessed restraints and skin integrity every 30 minutes.
- Discharged restraints at least every 2 hours.
- Appraised the need for restraints for every 4-8 hours.
- Stopped the restraint and applied the exercises on the limb and changed the position for there was cyanosis and pallor, coldness of a skin area.

Mrs. A has been still unconscious, aphasic and agitated, and continues to physically restraint on right wrists and ankles. She was discharged on bed from neurosurgery intensive care units after 35 days. Physical restraint has been still applied at your home. Mrs. A has a stage II pressure ulcers on coccyx and abrasion and edema on your wrist and ankle.

8. Conclusion

Physical restraint may be highly associated with nurses' monitoring and patients may suffer serious complications. Enhancements in intensive and acute care settings and in nurse staffing and education are necessary. Like many people, we believe that using physical restraint to control disruptive patient behaviors before alternative methods are tried or to compensate for shortages in nursing staff is unethical and unacceptable. In these conditions, use of physical restraints is an anathema to best practice principles, a denial of patient autonomy and beneficent professional health care practice principles. Nurses first have to consider patients' requests and needs if they wish to provide optimal care for patients/relatives.

Professional nursing practice accepts that the use of physical restraints is occasionally unnecessary, harmful, and potentially deadly (Demir 2007a,). Physical restraint used by nurses sometimes violates patients' autonomy or self respect and causes patients to lose their trust to the nurses. One should agree that physical restraint is an unethical assault on patients' rights and should be used carefully after alternative methods are tried (Demir-Zencirci-2009).

If physical restraint is used without enough care, it might result in life-threatening conditions, some of which were reported by respondents. Therefore, physical restraint without consent should not be used without physician orders or expert consultation. Last but not the least; nurses have always to remember that their responsibility is to offer optimal care to society and humankind, and best care to patients.

9. References

American Nurses Association. (2001). Ethics and Human Rights Position Statements: Reduction of Patient Restraint and Seclusion in Health Care Settings. Available at: http://www.nursingworld.org/MainMenuCategories/EthicsStandards/Ethics-Position-Statements/prtetrestrnt14452.aspx (accessed 27 July 2011).

Andanda, P. (2005). Module two: informed consent. Dev World Bioeth, 5:14- 29, ISSN 1471-8847

Arbesman, M.C. & Wright, C. (1999). Mechanical restraints, rehabilitation therapies, and staffing adequacy as risk factors for falls in an elderly hospitalised population. Rehabilitation Nursing, 24, 122–128, ISSN

Aveyard, H. (2005). Informed consent prior to nursing care procedures. Nurs Ethics,12:19-29, ISSN 0969-7330

Balon, J. A. (2001). Common factors of spontaneous self-extubation in a critical care setting. International Journal of Trauma Nursing, 7 (3), 93-99. ISSN: 1075-4210

Bandman, E.L. & Bandman, B. (2002). Ethical Issues in the Nursing Care of Elderly. *Nursing Ethics Through the Life Span*. (4th ed). London: Prentice- Hall International, p.233-59, ISSN 0-8385-6976-5

Beauchamp, T.L. & Childress, J.F. (2001). Moral Theories. *Principles of Biomedical Ethics*. (5th ed.) New York: Oxford University Pres, p: 337-77, ISSN 0-19-514332-9

Birkett, K.M.; Southerland, K.A. & Leslie, G.D. (2005). Reporting unplanned extubation. *Intensive Crit Care Nurs*,21:65-75; ISSN 0964-3397

Bonner, G.; Lowe, T.; Rawcliffe, D. & Wellman, N. (2002). Trauma for all: A pilot study of the subjective experience of physical restraint for mental health inpatients and staff in the UK. *Journal of Psychiatric and Mental Health Nursing*, 9, 465–473. ISSN 1351-0126

Bower, F.L. & McCullough, C.S. (2000). Restraint use in acute care settings: Can it be reduced? *Journal of Nursing Administration*, 30, 592–598, ISSN 0002-0443

Bray, K.; Hill, K.; Robson, W.; Leaver, G.; Walker, N.; O'Leary, M.; Delaney, T.; Walsh, D.; Gager, M. & Waterhouse, C. (2004). British association of critical care nurses position statement on the use of restraint in adult critical care units. *Nursing in Critical Care*; 9: 199–211. ISSN: 1478-5153.

Bridgman, A.M. & Wilson, M.A. (2000). The treatment of adult patients with mental disability. Part 1: Consent and duty. *British Dental Journal*, 189: 66-8, ISSN: 0007-0610

Burns, N. & Grove, S.K. (1999). Examining Ethics in Nursing Research. In: Understanding Nursing Research. 3rd ed. Philadelphia: WB Saunders Co, p: 159-92, ISSN 0-7216-0011-5

Calder, J. & Kirby, R.L. (1990). Fatal wheelchair-related accidents in the United States. *American Journal of Physical Medicine and Rehabilitation*, 69, 184–190, ISSN 0894-9115

Cannon, M.E.; Sprivulis, P. & McCarthy, J. (2001). Restraint practices in Australasian emergency departments. *Australian and New Zealand Journal of Psychiatry*, 35, 464–467, ISSN 0004-8674

Carrion, M.I.; Ayuso, D.; Marcos, M.; Robles, M.P.; De La Cal, M.A.; Alia, I. & Esteban, A. (2000). Accidental removal of endotracheal and nasogastric tubes and intravascular catheters. *Critical Care Medicine*, 28: 63–66. ISSN: 0090-3493

Castle, N.G. & Mor, V. (1987). Physical Restraints in Nursing Homes: A Review of the Literature Since the Nursing Home Reform Act of 1987. *Medical Care Research and Review*, 55: 139-170, ISSN: 1077-5587

Castle, N.G. (2002). Nursing homes with persistent deficiency citations for physical restraint use. *Medical Care*, 40: 868–878, ISSN 0025-7079

Choi, E. & Song, M. (2003). Physical restraint use in a Korean ICU. Journal of Clinical Nursing, 12, 651–659. ISSN: 0962-1067

Clary, G. & Krishnan, R. (2001). Delirium: Diagnosis, neuropath genesis and treatment. *Journal of Psychiatric Practice*, 7, 310–323, ISSN 1527-4160

Cohen, I.L.; Gallagher, T. J.; Pohlman, A.S.; Dasta, J.F.; Abraham, E. & Papadokos, P.J. (2002). Management of the agitated intensive care unit patient. *Critical Care Medicine*, 30 (suppl.): S97-S123, ISSN 0090-3493

Cruz, V.; Abdul-Hamid, M., Heater, B. (1997). Research-based practice: reducing restraints in an acute care setting – phase I, *Journal of Gerontological Nursing*, 23: 31-40, ISSN 0098-9134

Cull, C. & Inwood, H. (1999). Weaning patients from mechanical ventilation. *Professional Nurse*, 14: 535–538, ISSN 0266-8130

Currie, H.H. (1997). Cruel and unusual? The implications of section 12 of the Canadian charter of rights and freedoms on restraint use in care facilities. *Unpublished Master of Arts Thesis*. Simon Fraser University, Burnaby, BC, Canada.

Demir, A. (2007a). Nurses' Use of Physical Restraints in Four Turkish Hospitals, *Journal of Nursing Scholarship*, 39: 38-45, ISSN: 1527-6546

Demir, A. (2007b). The Use of Physical Restraints on Children: Practices and Attitudes of Paediatric Nurses in Turkey, *International Nursing Review*, 54: 367-374, ISSN 0020-8132

Demir-Zencirci, A. (2009). Attitudes, informed consent obtaining rates and feelings about physical restraint use among nurses, *Turkiye Klinikleri Journal of Medical Sciences*, 29:1571-1581, ISSN 1300-0292

Department of Constitutional Affairs. (2005). Mental Capacity Act. http://www.dca.gov.uk/menincap/legis.htm (accessed 20/01/06).

Department of Health and Welsh Office. (1999). Mental Health Act 1983 Code of Practise. London: Department of Health.

Department of Health. (2001). Reference Guide to Consent for Examination or Treatment. London: Department of Health.

Dimond, B. (2004). *Legal Aspects of Nursing*, 4rd edn. London: Longman, ISSN 0582822785

Doyal, L. (2001). Informed consent: moral necessity or illusion? *Qual Saf Health Care*,10(Suppl I):i29-i33, ISSN 2044-5415

Ely, E.W.; Margolin, R.; Francis, J.; May, L.; Truman, B.; Dittus, R.; Speroff, T.; Gautam, S.; Bernard, G.R. & Inouye, S.K. (2001). Evaluation of delirium in critically ill patients: validation of the confusion assessment method for the intensive care unit (CAM-ICU). *Critical Care Medicine*, 29: 1370-1379, ISSN 0090-3493

English, V.; Romano-Critchley, G.; Sheather, J. & Sommerville, A. (2004). Treatment without Consent: Incapacitated Adults and Compulsory Treatment. Medical Ethics Today The BMA's Handbook of Ethics and Law. 2nd ed. London, BMJ Publishing Group, p:99-126, ISBN: 978-0-7279-1744-7

Evans, D.; Wood, J. & Lambert, L. (2003). Patient injury and physical restraint devices: A systematic review. *Journal of Advanced Nursing*, 41: 274-282, ISSN 0309-2402

Evans, D.; Wood, J., Lambert, L. & FitzGerald, M. (2002). Physical restraint in acute and residential care: A systematic review. Adelaide, Australia: *The Joanna Briggs Institute.*

Fletcher, K. (1996). Use of Restraints in the Elderly. *AACN Clinical Issues*, 7: 611-620, ISSN 15597768

Frengley, J. D. & Mion, L. C. (1986). Incidence of physical restraints on acute general medical wards. *Journal of the American Geriatrics Society*, 34: 565-568, ISSN 1532-5415

Hamers, J.P.H. & Huizing, A.R. (2005). Why do we use physical restraints in the elderly? *Zeitschrift für Gerontologie und Geriatrie*, 38:19-25, ISSN 0948-6704

Happ, M. B. (2000). Preventing treatment interference: the nurse's role in maintaining technologic devices. *Heart and Lung*, 29: 60-69, ISSN: 0147-9563

Harrison, C.; Kenny, N.P.; Sidarous, M. & Rowell, M. (1997). Bioethics for clinicians: 9. Involving children in medical decisions. *CMAJ*,156(6):825-8, ISSN 0820-3946

Haskell, R.B.; Frankel, H.L. & Rotondo, M.F. (1997). Agitation. *AACN Clinical Issues*; 8: 335-350, ISSN 1079-0713

Hem, E.; Steen, O. & Opjordsmoen, S. (2001). Thrombosis associated with physical restraints. *Acta Psychiatrica Scandinavica*, 103, 73-76, ISSN 0001-690X

Hine, K. (2007). The use of physical restraint in critical care. *Nursing in critical care*, 12: 6-11, ISSN 1478-5153

HMSO. (1998). Human Rights Act. London: HMSO, ISSN 0-10-544298-4.

International Council of Nurses. The ICN code of ethics for nurses. *Nurs Ethics* 2001;8(4): 375-9, ISSN 0969-7330

Jensen, B.; Hess-Zak, A.; Johnston, S.K.; Otto, D.C.; Tebbe, L.; Russell, C. & Waller, A. (1998). Restraint reduction: A new philosophy for a new millenium. *Journal of Nursing Administration*, 28: 32-38, ISSN 0002-0443

Kanerva, A.M.; Suominen, T.& Leino-Kilpi H. (1999). Informed consent for short-stay surgery. *Nurs Ethics*, 6:483-93, ISSN 0969-7330

Kapp, M.B. (1996). Physical restraint use in critical care: legal issues. *AACN Clinical Issues*; 7: 579-584, ISSN 1079-0713

Koch, S. & Lyon, C. (2001). Case study approach to removing physical restraint. *International Journal of Nursing Practice*, 7:156-161, ISSN 1322-7114

Kozier, B.; Erb, G.; Berman, A. & Snyder, S. (2004). Safety. In, *Fundamentals of nursing* (7th ed.) Upper Saddle River, NJ: Prentice Hall, ISSN 0-13-114229

Lee, D.T.F.; Chan, M.C.; Tam, E.P.Y. & Yeung, W.S.K. (1999). Use of physical restraints on elderly patients: An exploratory study of the perceptions of nurses in Hong Kong. *Journal of Advanced Nursing*, 29, 153-159, ISSN 0309-2402

Ljunggren, G.; Phillips, C. & Sgadari, A. (1997). Comparisons of restraint use in nursing homes in eight countries. *Age and Ageing*, 16, 43-47, ISSN 0002-0729

Lofgren, R. P.; MacPherson, D. S.; Granieri, R.; Myllenbeck, S. & Sprafka, J. M. (1989). Mechanical restraints on the medical wards: Are protective devices safe? *American Journal of Public Health*, 79, 735-738, ISSN 0090-0036

Maccioli, G.A.; Dorman,T. & Brown, B.R. (2003). Clinical practice guidelines for the maintenance of patient physical safety in the intensive care unit: Use of restraining therapies—American College of Critical Care Medicine Task Force 2001-2002. *Critical Care Medicine*, 31: 2665-2676, ISSN 0090-3493

Macpherson, D.S.; Lofgren, R.P.; Cranieri, R. & Myllenbeck, S. (1990). Deciding to restrain medical patients. *Journal of the American Geriatrics Society*, 38,516-520, ISSN: 0002-8614

Martin, B. (2002). Restraint use in acute and critical care settings: changing practice. *AACN Clinical Issues*; 13: 294-306, ISSN 1079-0713

Minnick, A.F.; Mion, L.C.; Leipzig, R.; Lamb, K. & Palmer, R. (1998). Prevalence and patterns of physical restraint use in the acute care setting. *Journal of Nursing Administration*, 28: 19-24. ISSN 0002-0443

Mion, L. (1996). Establishing alternatives to physical restraint in the acute care setting: a conceptual framework to assist nurses' decision making. *AACN Clinical Issues*, 7: 592-602, ISSN 1079-0713

Mion, L. C.; Frengley, J. D.; Jakovcic, C. A. & Marino, J. A. (1989). A further exploration of the use of physical restraints in hospitalized patients. *Journal of the American Geriatrics Society*, 37, 949-956, ISSN 1532-5415

Moore, K. & Haralambous, B. (2007). Barriers to reducing the use of restraints in residential elder care facilities, *JAN*, 58(6), 532-540, ISSN 0309-2402

Morrison, A. (1997). Device errors. Incorrect restraint use: Deadly protection. *Nursing*, 27: 32, ISSN 0360-4039

Moss, R.J. & La Puma, J. (1991). The ethics of mechanical restraints. *Hastings Cent Rep*, 21:22-5, ISSN 0093-0334

Mott, S.; Poole, J. & Kenrick, M. (2005). Physical and chemical restraints in acute care: Their potential impact on the rehabilitation of older people. *International Journal of Nursing Practice*, 11, 95-101, ISSN 1322-7114

Nirmalan, M., Dark, P.M.; Nightingale, P. & Harris, J. (2004). Physical and pharmacological restraint of critically ill patients: clinical facts and ethical considerations. *British Journal of Anaesthesia*, 92: 789-792, ISSN 0007-0912

Paterson, B.; Bradley, P.; Stark, C.; Saddler, D.; Leadbetter, D. & Allen, D. (2003). Restraint related deaths in health social care in UK: Learning the lessons. *Mental Health Practice*, 6, 10-17,

Reay, D.T. (1998). Death in custody. *Clinics in Laboratory Medicine*, 18, 1-22, ISSN 0272-2712

Reigle, J. (1996). The ethics of physical restraints in critical care. *AACN Clinical Issues*, 7: 585–591, ISSN 1079-0713

Retsas, A.P. & Crabbe, H. (1998). Use of physical restraints in nursinghomes in New South Wales, Australia. *International Journal of Nursing Studies*, 35, 177–183, ISSN 0020-7489

Robbins, L. J.; Boyko, E.; Lane, J.; Cooper, D. & Jahnigen, D. W. (1987). Binding older persons: A prospective study of the use of mechanical restraints in an acute care hospital. *Journal of the American Geriatrics Society*, 35, 290-296.949-956, ISSN 1532-5415

Roberts, B. L. (2001). Managing delirium in intensive care patients. *Critical Care Nurse*, 21: 48-54, ISSN 0279-5442

Royal College of Nursing. (2004). Complementary therapies in nursing, midwifery and health visiting practice. RCN guidance on integrating complementary therapies into critical care. London: Author, Publication code 002 204

Sanders KM, Stern TA, O'Gara PT, Field TS, Rauch SL, Lipson RE, Eagle KA. (1992). Delirium during intra-aortic balloon pump therapy. Incidence and Management. Psychosomatics; 33: 35–44. ISSN 0033-3182

Shorr, R.I.; Guillen, M.K.; Rosenblaff, L.C.; Walker, K.; Caudle, C.E. & Kritchevsky, S.B. (2002). Restraint use, restraints orders, and the risk of falls in hospitalized patients. *Journal of the American Geriatrics Society*, 50, 526–529, ISSN 0002-8614

Stratton, S.J.; Rogers, C. & Brickett, K. (2001). Factors associated with sudden death in individuals requiring restraint for excited delirium. *American Journal of Emergency Medicine*, 19, 187– 191, ISSN 0735-6757

Sullivan-Marx, E.M.; Strumpf, N.E.; Evans, L.K.; Baumgarten, M. & Mailsin, G. (1999). Predictors of continued physical restraint use in nursing home residents following restraint reduction efforts. *Journal of the American Geriatrics Society*, 47, 342–348, ISSN 1532-5415

Swauger, K.C. & Tomlin, C.C. (2000). Moving toward restraint-free patient care. *Journal of Nursing Administration*, 30: 325–329, ISSN 0002-0443

Taylor, C.; Lillis, C. & LeMone, P. (1997). Safety. In, Fundamentals of nursing (3rd ed.; pp. 525–554). Philadelphia: Lippincott.

The General Directorate of Development of Regulations and Publishing. Patients' Rights Regulations. TC Resmi Gazete 1998;23420: 67-76.

Turkish Medical Association. (1999). Medicine and professional ethics. *Tıp Dünyası* 45:1-2:(col 1-7).

U.S. Department of Health and Human Services. (1984). Use of restraints: Federal standards. Washington, DC: Author.

Usher, K.J. & Arthur, D. (1998). Process consent: a model for enhancing informed consent in mental health nursing. *J Adv Nurs*, 27:692-7, ISSN: 0309-2402

Van Norman, G. & Palmer, S. (2001). The ethical boundaries of persuasion: Coercion and restraint of patients in clinical anaesthesia practice. *International Anaesthesiology Clinical*, 39, 131–143, ISSN: 0952-8180

Walker, L., Porter, M., Gruman, C. & Michalski, M. (1999). Developing Individualized Care in Nursing Homes: Integrating the Views of Nurses and Certified Nurse Aides. *Journal of Gerontological Nursing*, 25: 30-5, ISSN: 0098-9134

Westcott, C. (1995). The sedation of patients in intensive care units: a nursing review. *Intensive and Critical Care Nursing*, 11: 26-31, ISSN 0964-3397

Woodrow, P. & Roe, J. (2006). Intensive Care Nursing: A framework for practice. London: Routledge, ISSN: 0-415-37322-0

World Health Organization. (1994). A Decleration on the Promotion of Patients' Rights in Europe. European Consultation on the Rights of Patients. Amsterdam: WHO Regional Office for Europe, p:10-17.

Permissions

The contributors of this book come from diverse backgrounds, making this book a truly international effort. This book will bring forth new frontiers with its revolutionizing research information and detailed analysis of the nascent developments around the world.

We would like to thank Francesco Signorelli, for lending his expertise to make the book truly unique. He has played a crucial role in the development of this book. Without his invaluable contribution this book wouldn't have been possible. He has made vital efforts to compile up to date information on the varied aspects of this subject to make this book a valuable addition to the collection of many professionals and students.

This book was conceptualized with the vision of imparting up-to-date information and advanced data in this field. To ensure the same, a matchless editorial board was set up. Every individual on the board went through rigorous rounds of assessment to prove their worth. After which they invested a large part of their time researching and compiling the most relevant data for our readers. Conferences and sessions were held from time to time between the editorial board and the contributing authors to present the data in the most comprehensible form. The editorial team has worked tirelessly to provide valuable and valid information to help people across the globe.

Every chapter published in this book has been scrutinized by our experts. Their significance has been extensively debated. The topics covered herein carry significant findings which will fuel the growth of the discipline. They may even be implemented as practical applications or may be referred to as a beginning point for another development. Chapters in this book were first published by InTech; hereby published with permission under the Creative Commons Attribution License or equivalent.

The editorial board has been involved in producing this book since its inception. They have spent rigorous hours researching and exploring the diverse topics which have resulted in the successful publishing of this book. They have passed on their knowledge of decades through this book. To expedite this challenging task, the publisher supported the team at every step. A small team of assistant editors was also appointed to further simplify the editing procedure and attain best results for the readers.

Our editorial team has been hand-picked from every corner of the world. Their multi-ethnicity adds dynamic inputs to the discussions which result in innovative outcomes. These outcomes are then further discussed with the researchers and contributors who give their valuable feedback and opinion regarding the same. The feedback is then collaborated with the researches and they are edited in a comprehensive manner to aid the understanding of the subject.

Apart from the editorial board, the designing team has also invested a significant amount of their time in understanding the subject and creating the most relevant covers. They scrutinized every image to scout for the most suitable representation of the subject and create an appropriate cover for the book.

The publishing team has been involved in this book since its early stages. They were actively engaged in every process, be it collecting the data, connecting with the contributors or procuring relevant information. The team has been an ardent support to the editorial, designing and production team. Their endless efforts to recruit the best for this project, has resulted in the accomplishment of this book. They are a veteran in the field of academics and their pool of knowledge is as vast as their experience in printing. Their expertise and guidance has proved useful at every step. Their uncompromising quality standards have made this book an exceptional effort. Their encouragement from time to time has been an inspiration for everyone.

The publisher and the editorial board hope that this book will prove to be a valuable piece of knowledge for researchers, students, practitioners and scholars across the globe.

List of Contributors

Pratipal Kalsi and David Choi
National Hospital for Neurology & Neurosurgery, London, United Kingdom

Luca Arpino and Pierpaolo Nina
Department of Neurosurgery, San Giovanni Bosco Hospital, Naples, Italy

H. Selim Karabekir
Department of Neurosurgery, Kocatepe University School of Medicine, Afyonkarahisar, Turkey

Nuket Gocmen-Mas
Department of Anatomy, Faculty of Medicine, Kocatepe University, Afyonkarahisar, Turkey

Mete Edizer
Department of Anatomy, Faculty of Medicine, Dokuz Eylul University, Izmir, Turkey

Dirk Winkler, Marc Tittgemeyer, Karl Strecker, Axel Goldammer, Jochen Helm, Johannes Schwarz and Jürgen Meixensberger
Department of Neurosurgery, University of Leipzig, Leipzig, Germany

Antonio Daniele, Pietro Spinelli and Chiara Piccininni
Istituto di Neurologia, Università Cattolica, Rome, Italy

Shuxiang Guo, Jian Guo, Nan Xiao and Takashi Tamiya
Kagawa University, Japan

E.O. Vik-Mo, A. Fayzullin, M.C. Moe, H. Olstorn and I.A. Langmoen
Vilhelm Magnus Laboratory, Department of Neurosurgery and Institute of Surgical Research, Oslo University Hospital, Norway

Tapio Heikkilä, Pekka Kilpeläinen and Mikko Sallinen
VTT Technical Research Centre of Finland, Finland

Sanna Yrjänä and John Koivukangas
Department of Neurosurgery, University of Oulu, Oulu, Finland

F. Lapierre, S. D'Houtaud and M. Wager

Ayten Demir Zencirci
Ankara University, Faculty of Health Sciences, Nursing Department, Turkey

Printed in the USA
CPSIA information can be obtained
at www.ICGtesting.com
JSHW011415221024
72173JS00004B/548